J. Rutter (John Rutter) Williamson

The healing of the nations

A Treatise on Medical Missions, Statement and Appeal.

J. Rutter (John Rutter) Williamson

The healing of the nations
A Treatise on Medical Missions, Statement and Appeal.

ISBN/EAN: 9783741169113

Manufactured in Europe, USA, Canada, Australia, Japa

Cover: Foto ©Andreas Hilbeck / pixelio.de

Manufactured and distributed by brebook publishing software
(www.brebook.com)

J. Rutter (John Rutter) Williamson

The healing of the nations

The Healing of the Nations

A Treatise on Medical Missions
Statement and Appeal

BY J. RUTTER WILLIAMSON

(M.B., Edinburgh University)

Traveling Secretary Student Volunteer Movement
Late Chairman British Student Volunteer Missionary Union
Member of British Medical Association

Καὶ τοῦ ποταμοῦ ἐντεῦθεν καὶ ἐκεῖθεν ξύλον ζωῆς ποιοῦν καρποὺς δώδεκα, κατὰ μῆνα ἕκαστον ἀποδιδοῦν τὸν καρπὸν αὐτοῦ, καὶ τὰ φύλλα τοῦ ξύλου εἰς θεραπείαν τῶν ἐθνῶν.—Rev, xxii. 2.

NEW YORK
STUDENT VOLUNTEER MOVEMENT FOR FOREIGN MISSIONS

TO

MY MOTHER

WHOSE CONSTANT AND ENDURING INTEREST IN

THE WORK OF

WORLD-WIDE MISSIONS

TOUCHED MY CHILDISH FANCIES

STIRRED THE IMAGINATION OF MY BOYISH YEARS

AND

DEEPENED THE PURPOSES OF MY MANHOOD

IS THIS LITTLE BOOK

AFFECTIONATELY DEDICATED

BY HER SON

PREFACE

This little volume has been written primarily to provide an outline of Medical Missions, for the use of students and young people in Missionary Study Classes. There has also been kept in mind the far larger circle of Christian people whose interest in the work of Missionary Medicine has been limited by their scanty information on the subject. It is not such a book as would be read aloud, for instance, at a women's sewing meeting, but it is rather intended for study and individual perusal. Its aim is to present facts that ought to be pondered in the hearts of Christian men and women in the Church of Christ, and the subject makes a special claim upon the consideration of those who are members of the medical and nursing professions.

There is no classic on Medical Missions, unless we except the Gospels.* There is need of one. No one, for instance, has, as far as we are aware, worked out at all fully the psychological aspects of the subject. In the standard works on psychology, we have been able to discover but little dealing with the psychology of the religious emotions which were generated in the hearts of men and women through the touch of Christ. Artists and poets, with their intuitive perceptions, almost always tell of personal contact between the Saviour and those healed. Though not apparently bearing much on the actual claims that suffering makes on the medical profession, this would

---

* The nearest approximation to a classic is, possibly, "Medical Missions: Their Place and Power," by Dr. John Lowe.

be at least an interesting as well as a valuable scientific contribution to the subject.

Somewhat more has appeared in the realm of Sociology and the wider influence upon public life that Medical Missions have had. Dr. James S. Dennis's unsurpassed work on " Christian Missions and Social Progress " gives an important section to the consideration of this topic. There is great need for some work which would co-ordinate the fast accumulating material on Medical Missions in periodical literature, and marshal its principles and practices into a harmonious whole.

As a text-book, this is necessarily but a meager outline of the subject. The argument from Scripture we have taken for granted throughout. It is a topic which has received generous treatment at the hands of other writers, and therefore did not seem to demand the emphasis that has been laid on other less frequently noticed aspects.

Our warmest thanks are due to Dr. James S. Dennis for his valuable assistance and suggestions as well as for permission to use the statistics given on page eighty-nine.

J. R. W.

NEW YORK, JUNE 1, 1899.

CONTENTS

ARGUMENT FOR MEDICAL MISSIONS

"I am in earnest ; I will not equivocate, I will not excuse. I will not retreat a single inch and I will be heard."
—William Lloyd Garrison.

"My country is the world. My countrymen are all mankind."
—William Lloyd Garrison.

"The world's a room of sickness, where each heart
Knows its own anguish and unrest ;
The truest wisdom there and noblest art
Is his who skills of comfort best."
—Keble.

"I have long since ceased to pray ' Lord Jesus, have compassion on a lost world.' I remember the day and the hour when I seemed to hear the Lord rebuking me for making such a prayer. He seemed to say to me, ' I have had compassion upon a lost world and now it is time for you to have compassion. I have left you to fill up that which is wanting in Mine afflictions in the flesh for the body's sake, which is the Church. I have given My heart ; now give your hearts.' "
—A. J. Gordon.

"The student of social philosophy in determining the stage of civilization at which any nation has arrived regards as an almost infallible criterion the degree of esteem in which its women are held."
—Edward Balfour.

THE HEALING OF THE NATIONS

I

ARGUMENT FOR MEDICAL MISSIONS

Foreword. An old church in Damascus which was built in the early days of Christianity, had the words " To the Glory of God," inscribed over the portal. The Muhammedans captured it and plastered it over. Now the plaster has fallen and revealed the old inscription. In the spring days of the Christian Era deeds of mercy to the sick were counted part of the life of love which the Lover of Men had infused into His followers.

These kindly offices to those stricken in body have ever been a glory of Christianity. Though sometimes in the clash and clangor of doctrinal strife the Church has well nigh forgotten its ministry to the sick, yet its neglect has been but for a little season, to be renewed by at least some select and holy souls, with greater fervency and devotion.

The association of Religion and Medicine is perfectly natural. The Christian religion claims to complete and consummate, as well as to comprehend, the ends of Medicine. A God is only thinkable in terms of everlasting life. " We are the ministers of life. He is the Prince of Life. We fight against death and are all defeated. Death assailed Him and He vanquished death." In this fight for length of life He is not ashamed to call us brethren. The justification of the marriage between healing and preaching is the life of Christ. It was reserved for these closing days of the second thousand years of Christianity to revive on a comparatively large scale the work of treating the sick, in demonstration of the love of God toward their bodies as well as souls. In no sphere is this demonstration more needed than among those who have never yet heard the story of the Healer of Men. To

7

the heathen abroad, as well as to the godless at home, the most convincing proof of the love of God is that it begets love to man.

Definition. By a Medical Missionary we mean one who takes the fruits of the Christian Era as exemplified in modern Medicine and thus seeks to plant the roots of Christianity in nations and among peoples who are ignorant of its doctrines. The Medical Mission is, as Dr. Willard Parker used to say, Clinical Christianity. The late professor of medicine in Oxford University said recently in speaking on Medical Missions, "that any religion to be true must be such as would appeal to all men of every race, and in any period of its evolution," and that the religion of Jesus exemplified in the work of the Medical Missionary did this pre-eminently.

Purpose. The purpose of Medical Missions is not simply philanthropic, though it finds its glory in self-sacrificing philanthropy. It is not merely an enterprise to secure the inestimable benefits of Western Medicine and Surgery for those in these terribly needy lands. Its purpose is not educative alone, though its educational influences are far-reaching; nor is it to provide a temporal benefit as a bribe for spiritual blessing.

The purpose of Medical Missions is to win men to Jesus Christ by the use of methods precisely comparable to those used by Christ when on earth, as the Great Succorer of Bodies, as well as Divine Saviour of Souls.

Necessity for Consideration. It is passing strange that attention should need to be drawn to the sweet influences of this love-work. It would have seemed so natural a deduction from the religion of which love is the essence, even if we had not the records of Christ's example.

> "As every lovely hue is light,
>   So every grace is love,"

and this sphere of service is surely one in which real abiding love to fellow-men can be more impressively shown than in almost any other.

Yet to-day its privilege and duty is by no means unquestioned. The very fact that North America and Britain have two hundred and thirty times as many physicians as there are Medical Missionaries among the whole of heathendom, is ample proof that the Church has not yet begun to realize the claims of those other lands for loving medical attention. The united population of these two countries is but one-ninth of the heathen world. Can it be that such a population requires 156,000 physicians and can spare less than 700 for the neglected one thousand millions in mission lands?

Love is the distinguishing characteristic of the Christian religion. Other teachers had set high standards of faith, others had preached the sternest self-sacrifice; some had even attempted to shadow forth a high hope in the future; but Christ alone among the great masters has placed this quality as the test of discipleship, and as the manifestation of the Godhead. " By this," we hear Him say, " By this shall all men know that ye are MY disciples, if ye have love one to another." Not only has this been recognized by students of comparative religions; it is recognized by the world. The world cares little about the exercise of faith by professing Christians. It frankly confesses its inability to comprehend faith. As to hope, it allows the Church to please itself about its glorious hope of a hereafter, but when it comes to love, it is keen to observe and mark every breach.

If we are to follow in the steps of Jesus, it is not optional, but essential, that we walk even as He walked, in the path of love. As the justification for Medical Missions is the career of Christ, so the prime motive for their prosecution is love toward Christ and through Him toward men.

The Argument for Medical Missions. The argument for Medical Missions is manifold. We see it expressed by the appalling need for such work in the lands under consideration. This need is seen in the ignorance displayed by those professing to be the physicians of these people.

Ignorance. The native doctors are absolutely ignorant of the rudiments of scientific medicine. The first thing an embryonic medical student in China does is to commit to memory the three hundred places in the body through which skewers may be driven with safety. Some of these so-called " safe " places are actually through the abdomen and lungs!

It is strange in a country like China, for instance, where critical examinations attend each step of a literary degree, that no test of any sort is demanded from those who practice medicine. There are no doctors in our sense of the word—men who have studied the science and received the imprimatur of some examining body. Many of the native doctors are those who have failed in the literary examinations, or who have been unfortunate in business.

They divide diseases into " outside," or surgical, and " inside," or medical cases. A doctor's sign often bears the legend, " Outside and inside diseases cured." Their knowledge of anatomy is still practically nil. No dissections are permitted in the Empire. A copper model with imaginary organs in imaginary places is sometimes used for instruction. They are wholly innocent of any such fine distinctions as the differences between veins, arteries, nerves and tendons. The trachea is two inches wide and one foot long. The liver has seven lobes and is the motor centre for the eyes and also contains the soul. The larynx goes through the lungs directly to the heart. The centre of the thorax is the seat from which joy and delight emanate. No Harvey has yet arisen to teach the Chinese the laws of the circulation of the blood. Authors vary a good deal in their views. Some " represent tubes issuing from the fingers and toes and running up the limbs into the trunk, where they are lost or reach the heart, lungs, or some other organ as well as they can, wandering over most parts of the body in their course." The Chinese know nothing of the nervous system, its functions or its diseases. The position of the heart is stated to be midway between the crown of the head and the sole of the foot—" it must be there," is the logical explanation, " for it's the centre of the being."

The pharmacopœia of these lands is remarkable. Both in Persia and China remedies are divided into hot and cold. When refrigerants have failed for a long time they will say: " Perhaps the patient has had too much of it;

we will change the treatment and try something hot."
" One last resource remains to the Persian physician to
save his own reputation—to recommend the patient to try
a forty days' course of a decoction made from a certain
root. The victim must take it forty days consecutively,
three times a day, about half a pint at a time, after food,
and never once lose his or her temper, or it will be of no
avail. The fortieth day the patient returns probably
worse than before, or complains of feeling certainly none
the better, and at once the physician says, ' But have you
lost your temper?' Of course, he or she has, and then it
is not the physician's fault but the patient's."

A favorite remedy in Korea for anæmia is a jelly made
from the bones of a man recently killed. A criminal exe-
cution is largely attended by native practitioners to obtain this valuable ingredient. (The author has sometimes wondered if this betokened a sort of lucky foresight
into our modern treatment of some anæmias by adminis-
tration of bone-marrow!)

For catarrhs chips from coffins which have been let
down into the grave are boiled and said to possess great
virtue.

A medical missionary recently told a story of a man
who had come to him with dyspepsia. He had been ordered to take stone ground up in a paste with water.
During two years he had taken each day a cupful and
had consumed half a millstone, about sixty pounds in
weight. Finding himself no better, he was ordered cin-
namon bark and had ingested forty pounds of it. It
seems to us a great tribute to the man's constitution to
be able to record that ten days of more appropriate treatment resulted in his complete recovery in spite of the he-
roic measures previously employed!

According to Dr. Wells Williams some of the agents
administered are at once archaic and archeological. They
include snake skins, fossil bones, rhinoceros or hart's
horn shavings, silk worm and human secretions, asbestos,
moths and oyster shells. But this list is nothing to one
that was recorded in a recent Chinese medical missionary
journal: " Flies are of great use to man, for their heads
when pounded and used as a pomade form an infallible

hair restorer for the head, beard and eyebrows. . . .
Bats are harmless animals and of great value in medicine.
Their flesh, applied as a poultice, is a sovereign cure for
the stings of scorpions; roasted and eaten, they dry up
the excess of saliva in infants. . . . There is nothing
better for that dangerous disease, lethargy, than to put
fleas into the patient's ears." Speaking of bedbugs, "certain
devout and religious people have been known to put those
animals in their beds, that they might be more wakeful
to contemplate divine things. . . . One purpose of
their creation was, doubtless, to keep us from pride, . . .
but the main object of the creation of bugs was the benefit of the sick. They are of remarkable efficacy in the
hysteria of females, if one puts them in the patient's nose.
. . . Seven bugs taken in barley water are of great
value in quartan ague and for the bites of scorpions."
The writer who quotes the above adds, " Heaven has certainly been bountiful to China and well stocked Nature's
Dispensary."

In Korea the bones of a tiger are considered a specific
for cowardice. A strong tiger-bone soup will make a
hero of the most arrant coward. They argue thus: " The
tiger is very strong; his bones are the strongest part of
him, therefore a soup of the bones must be wonderfully
strengthening." For those who cannot afford such an
expensive luxury, they may yet obtain some of the
strength and courage of that ferocious beast by swallow-
ing a decoction of his mustache hairs, which are retailed
at the ridiculously low figure of one hundred cash—i.e., 3
to 6 cents—per hair!

Ophthalmia and other eye diseases are extremely common in almost all these lands. The author during a trip
to Palestine once noticed no fewer than ten different diseases of the eye in the course of a half hour's stroll
through the bazars of Jerusalem. Thousands become
sightless every year through the lack of the simplest lo-
tions and ointments. In China there are estimated to be
no fewer than 500,000 blind. and in India the number is
stated to be 458,000. Ophthalmia is still treated in many
places by a lotion of boiled monkey's feet, pork and alco-
hol, and notwithstanding such original treatment no cures

.re reported. A missionary in India describes the case
)f a child who was brought to her for eye treatment:
' The poor mother said, ' I have been so careful; I have
)ut the country medicine in each day.' We asked what
t was, and this was the answer : 'A donkey's tooth ground
ip with charcoal, and the powder put into the child's eyes.'
\nd for two whole months the mother had patiently ap-
)lied this."

Their knowledge of pathology is such that resinous
)lasters or dabs of tar are put on whenever pus appears.
f the suppuration burrows its way through, more plas-
er is applied. The ruling principle is to keep it in.

Some of these practices would be merely ludicrous if
t were not for the terrible suffering entailed by such absurd
reatment. A physician of the Celestial Empire does not
iesitate to thrust a long, uncleanly needle into a patient's
tomach or liver who comes to him suffering with dyspep-
ia. Add to this the custom of blistering the wounds
hus caused, and the extreme danger of the procedure will
)e realized.

Of course there must be here and there exceptions,
vhere the treatment prescribed is at least harmless and
)ccasionally beneficial. There is, however, no scientific
tudy of the subject, and there are none of the instru-
nents of precision for diagnosis which to-day are the
)roperty of the whole profession in our more favored
ountries. The stethoscope, clinical thermometer, micro-
cope and staining agents are of course quite unknown.

uperstition. Mrs. Isabella Bird-Bishop, the celebrated
Asiatic traveler, says that back of almost
all Asiatic religions is the belief in demons.
)emonism underlies the Indian religions; it is para-
nount in Afghanistan and in much of Arabia, and is the
)edrock on which the Taoism of China is built. If this
)e true of Asia, it is no less true of large parts of Africa.
.he demons need to be exorcised in cases of sickness.
.he first question is not, as with us, what is the cause of
his sickness, but rather, who is the cause. In Africa, the
nedicine man is called in to know who has bewitched
he sick one. He has a string of shells, and by throwing
hese in the air and watching how they fall he pretends

to know the exact man, or his spirit should he be dead.
It is vain for the selected one to protest his innocence.
" If a man has an apoplectic stroke, this is not due to the
rupture of a blood vessel in his brain or to any other of the
natural causes of this condition, but some enemy has cast
a spell over him or perhaps his father's ghost is angry
with him."

It is the natural result of such belief in witch-
craft that charms and spells should play an important part
in the treatment of disease. Clairvoyance, miraculous in-
terpositions and supernatural appearances are common-
places in the systems of belief in many parts of the
heathen world, and are constantly resorted to in times of
sickness. Fortune tellers and astrologers are protected
by law in China. In the recent Chinese war some interesting examples occurred of the superstitious darkness
which still hangs as a pall upon even the comparatively intelligent. A general whose arm was shattered by a ball,
thinking the daily dressing in Western style was too slow
a method, called in a fortune teller. Prayers were written in the picturesque Chinese characters upon red paper.
This was burnt and the ashes administered as medicine.
During four days the wound was left unattended and the
general died from blood poisoning.

In Persia during an epidemic of cholera, thousands of
prayers were printed and posted above the doors of the
houses. They were of various kinds; some in Arabic
gave detailed directions from the Angel Gabriel that who-
soever should write out this prayer and " keep it about his
person shall be safe, and whoever reads it once a day for
seven days, shall be exempt. And whoever shall write
it and put it in a cup of water, and shall drink of that
water, the disease of cholera shall not reach him." A
traveler in India passing through a village noticed that
decapitated dogs had been put up in trees at the various
entrances to the village. Those horrible sights were so
placed that from whichever side the Cholera Goddess
might approach, she might be turned back in disgust.

In China and India gongs are beaten and firecrackers
ignited to frighten away the evil spirits which are supposed to be the cause of the sickness. Such a scene is

vividly pictured by a missionary who witnessed the sight :
" Hearing the noise of a drum, I asked what it was, and
the woman told me it was a ' girl playing.' It seems she
had been very ill for two months, and as all remedies had
failed, the *hakim* (doctor) said she must be under the
power of an evil spirit. The ' magicians ' were sent for
to exorcise the demon. In a small, hot room was a crowd
of men, women and children ; in the middle, the two ' wizards '—leering men, with faces sodden with good living
and evil doing. One beat a drum, the other thumped
with brass pokers on a metal instrument. At intervals
they recited incantations. The patient was lying on the
ground before them, while a woman ironed her with a hot
brick. ' Lift her up,' said one of the ' wizards.' This
was done and then began a most sickening sight. She
writhed backward and forward like a snake being
charmed, the movements getting quicker and quicker as
the drums beat louder ; then she knocked her head and long
black hair upon the ground. I spoke to the mother, but
it was of no use, and the evil looking men beat the drum
more furiously than ever. In such places Satan's seat is
firm." Of course, such superstition is the avenue for
fraud and blackmail of a most exacting kind.

Fracture cases which have been treated with splints
in mission hospitals are often carried away by their
friends to have the splints removed and the fracture
smeared over with mud from some shrine, in the belief that
it will unite better.

In Palestine a missionary physician was called in to
see the son of a local governor. He found the native
" hakim " had written the word "Allah," the Arabic name
for God, round a plate and then washed it off, giving the
boy the inky draught. He was sure that he must recover
now that he had drunk the name of God so many times.

Bites by dogs are said to be best treated by drawing a
circle round the wound and writing the word " tiger " in
it, because the tiger is more than a match for the dog.

" The disease demons may afflict the patient in various
ways. They come behind him, and hitting him with a
club, enter the back of his neck, or creep into his
body and consume his liver. A spirit may get

into the body and 'gnaw and feed' inside; invisible
spirits may inflict invisible wounds with invisible spears,
or, lodging in the heart, may make men mad. Sometimes
it is the spirit of a bear, deer, turtle, fish, tree, stone or
worm sent into the spirit of the sick man, or, as we have
often heard them say, ' a ghost sitting on the chest of a
patient.' . . .
  " Thorns and bushes are put in the pathway of the smallpox spirit, or thorns, ditches and stinking oils may bar-
ricade the way of his approach. In New Zealand the
disease demon is to be charmed on a flag-staff; in Mala-
gasy the patient's ailments are to be recounted to some
grass, ashes, a sheep or a pumpkin, and the disease spirit
prayed to for their removal. The Patagonian was wont
to beat a drum and the Dacota to shake his gourd and
bead rattle to scare away the disease. The most widespread formula, however, is that of sucking or blowing on
the diseased organs, accompanied with incantations, and
the extraction of stones, splinters and bits of rags, amidst
drumming, dancing and drinking. Not infrequently
the disease is transferred by various means. The sick
man's blood may be run into an ant-hill or dropped in the
mouth of a frog or a live fowl, or sent into a leopard's
claw, a nail, a rag, a puppy or a duck. Such being the
world's theories of disease and its treatment, it is plain
that medicine and theology go together in the thought and
life of the non-Christian man. He is quite prepared to
receive them together from the Christian missionary.
' In nothing has the savage (and it is true of many more
than the savage) been more religious than in his medicine,
if it may be so called,' says one of the ablest ethnogra-
phers of our day. His medicine-man is always his priest,
whether we call him shaman, conjurer, sorcerer or wiz-
ard. Sickness being the effect of the anger of a god, or
the malicious influence of a sorcerer, he naturally seeks
relief from his deity. ' The recovery from disease is the
kindliest exhibition of Divine power, and the Christian
Medical Missionary occupies a lofty vantage ground in
his work.' "*
  Superstition is the subtlest and most tenacious enemy

*" Women's Medical Work in Foreign Lands," by Mrs. J. T. Gracey, pp. 10-12.

of Christianity. In no way can the belief in demons be more effectually shattered than by the work of the Medical Missionary. A minor operation, or a few doses of medicine, may cure a condition which has been affirmed to be consequent on some bewitching agency and which cannot be cured except by incantations, mantrams, or gaudy idolatrous processions to appease the wrath of some plague god, or disease demon.

It is difficult for those in Christian countries to realize the vast amount of suffering—mental and physical—which might be prevented and of sorrow which might be comforted, if only the voice of the Husbandman was heard as He calls for laborers to dress the vines and gather the grapes, which now are being so bruised and downtrodden in His far-away vineyards.

We would conclude this chapter by telling a story which is being enacted to-day in countless homes of India —a strange, weird mingling of ignorance, superstition, cruelty and neglect, which will surely appeal to the tenderness of every woman reader.

It is the home of a high-caste Hindu. A mother and a little child less than a week old are lying unconscious. The mother has survived the unspeakable barbarities of the native midwife, and now she and her child are perishing for want of food and from neglect.

" Every step of her treatment had been laid down in their sacred book. . . . For the first three days she has been deprived of food and drink, and on the third allowed one grain of rice. Her room has been prepared by placing her in the darkest and dirtiest of the house, with the most filthy of rags, on a mud floor for her bed. A cow's skull painted red, an image of Sasthi, the goddess who presides over the destiny of women and children, . . . is placed in a conspicuous position. This and the pot of smoldering charcoal, the only furniture, are placed there to expel the evil spirits hovering round. During her three weeks of uncleanness neither father, mother, husband nor sister can come nigh her, leaving her to the care of the barber's wife. On the fifth day the filthy clothing is removed and the room cleaned, as on the next is to be the worship of Sasthi, and that night Vidhata

will write on the child's forehead the main events of his
life.   The day has arrived, Sasthi has been worshiped.
The woman has been given a cold bath, all necessary ar-
rangements for Vidhata's visit have been made, food con-
sisting of a coarse graham flour and coarser brown sugar,
equal parts, wet and kneaded together, to be eaten raw,
has been prepared for the famished mother, but both
mother and child are unconscious, and the foreign doctor
is called to bring them back to life."*   These are thy
Gods, O India; these are Thy rivals, O Jehovah!

When shall a prophet of God be able to look toward
these dark places and chant the anthem, "Arise, shine, for
thy light is come, and the glory of the Lord is risen upon
thee"?

---

* *Missionary Review of the World*, September 1893, p. 688.

MALPRACTICE IN HEATHEN LANDS

" In the name of God, Who has made us of one blood and in Whose image we are created ; in the name of the Messiah Who came to bind up the broken hearted, to proclaim liberty to the captives and the opening of the prison to them that are bound, I demand the immediate emancipation of those who are pining."

—William Lloyd Garrison.

" Ask God to give thee skill
    In comfort's art,
  That thou may'st consecrated be
    And set apart
  Unto a life of sympathy.
  For heavy is the weight of ill
    In every heart,
  And comforters are needed much
  Of Christ-like touch."

—A. E. Hamilton.

" For the heart grows rich in giving : all its wealth is living grain.
  Seeds which mildew in the garner, scattered, fill with gold the plain.
  Is thy burden hard and heavy?   Do thy steps drag wearily ?
  Help to bear thy brother's burden : God will bear both it and thee."

—Mrs. Charles.

" The possession of a great ideal does not mean, as so many fondly imagine, work accomplished : it means work revealed—work revealed so vast, often so impossible, that faith and hope die down, and the enthusiast of yesterday becomes the cynic of to-morrow."

—George Adam Smith.

II

MALPRACTICE IN HEATHEN LANDS

It is stated that whenever Captain Cook touched new soil in his travels he sowed seeds of British plants. Later colonists found to their surprise plants of their home land growing in their newly adopted countries. As we voyage in thought along the shores of history we see that wherever Christianity has gone there grows more or less luxuriantly the flower of brotherly love—a veritable sensitive plant to rough and careless handling. It is a great thing for our lands to-day that the body politic is so exquisitely alive toward customs which involve pain or cruelty to either the lower animals or to fellow men. Sometimes this public conscience may seem to be callous for a while; sometimes it becomes morbid or hysterical; yet, as a whole, in every Christian nation, it is to be profoundly trusted to eventually deliver a right judgment. Cock-fighting, bull-baiting, pugilism, cruelty to helpless children, or to the blind or insane, are all doomed in every nation which seeks to follow even afar off in the steps of the Great Altruist.

The Christian world is a great nervous system which feels the shock and thrill of pain from its most distal extremities. Atrocities in Armenia, famines in India, floods in China, persecutions in Russia and misgovernment of degraded or oppressed peoples, all bring their message and make impact upon thought, memory, prayer—and at last, though, alas, slowly, stir the heart to help, rescue and redeem.

" He's true to God who's true to man wherever wrong is done
To the humblest and the weakest 'neath the all-beholding sun.
That wrong is also done to us, and they are slaves most base
Whose love of right is for themselves, and not for all their race."

Yet there seems to be a strange anæsthesia which has

settled upon the Church of Christ in reference to the bodily
pangs and pains which are being so agonizingly felt by
thousands for whom the temporal as well as spiritual bless-
ings of Christianity were intended. Is it that she has received these messages of pain so infrequently that a path
has hardly been established toward her perception centres,
or has she merely been slow to discern from whence they
came and to what duty they called her?

Whatever be the true reason, the fact is patent that the
followers of Christ have allowed this suffering to continue
unmitigated by loving help, and are only now beginning
to realize and rescue.

Cruelty. " The tender mercies of the wicked are cruel."
Ignorance in the treatment of the sick were bad
enough; superstition is degrading and paralyzing in its
effects; but cruelty blasts the dim light of conscience which
is in every man's secret heart and hardens the unhappy
victim into desperation and despair.

" In Arabia, an ingenious expedient for relieving a patient is burning holes in the body to let the disease out,
branding sick children with red hot bars, chopping off
wounded limbs and sealing them with boiling tar." Cut-
ting with knives and scarification are frequently resorted
to. Sometimes, of course, this violent counter-irritation
is of some benefit, at least temporarily, though the result-
ant wounds often suppurate for years after the operation.
A Chinese doctor has great faith in moxa, which is a powder made of various medicaments including saltpetre, and
which is ignited on the skin of the patient.

Dr. Rosetta S. Hall gives an account of the visit of a
Korean doctor to a sick child : " The first thing he did was
to make a little pyramid of brownish looking powder
upon each breast of the child, and then to set it on fire until it burned the tender skin. This was followed by the
use of a large darning needle, which was first thrust
through each little foot, then the palms of the hands, the
thumb joints, and through the lips into the jaw, just be-
neath the nose." Imagine, if you can, the agonizing
screams of the child while this barbarous and useless
cruelty was being practiced!

Think of the treatment in this land of mothers in the

throes of childbirth and compare it with the customs in heathen lands. Here, all is made subservient to the mother's comfort. If she is poor, our splendid maternity hospitals are open for her reception. The room is prepared, the footfall becomes more quiet as it approaches her door, the merry shouting of the children is hushed, friends are near, and the trained skill of nurse and physician are at her command. "All Hindu women," wrote the veteran missionary, Mrs. Weitbrecht, some few years since, " whether rich or poor, are utterly neglected in time of sickness." The native nurses are all the majority of sick women in India have for doctors. They are ignorant, immoral and excessively meddlesome. Countless mothers and infants fall a prey to horrible barbarities inflicted in the name of service, during their hour of peril. In India a tardy labor is assisted by a bamboo pole, or a plank of wood laid across the woman's abdomen, with a heavy assistant seated on each end. In Siam the mother is made to expose herself for many days to a fire built up of wood about eighteen inches from her body, with the result that serious burns occur, causing weeks or months of suffering, and at length healing with extensive cicatrices and the usual diseases consequent upon prolonged suppuration. Supposed to be possessed by some evil spirit, they are objects to be shunned, and every possible cruelty may be resorted to that the demon may be expelled. In some places the mother is banished in a winter cold, many degrees below zero, to a hut of bark for ten days, and is frequently quite alone and often half starved.

A lady missionary relates a visit she paid to the home of a Muhammedan teacher, where both wife and children are loved by husband and father. On the bed is a little child of three years in convulsions. "As we enter, a barber has just finished shaving the hair from the head just over . . . . the place where the brain can be seen to pulsate in an infant's head and is called by the natives of India ' the door to the brain.' A Muhammedan doctor lifts a red hot piece of iron from the fire and presses it to the exposed part, destroying the tissues to the skull, and to my cry of horror and dismay the father, in an agony of sorrow, answers, ' Oh, Miss Sahib, for many days that door was open and an evil spirit entered there and must be destroyed, or our child will die.' "

A dislocated ankle is reduced by strapping two boards to the sole of the foot and driving a stout wedge between them, much on the same principle as the infamous " boot " used during the Inquisition.

Fractures are sometimes placed in splints of rough unpadded bark and are tied up with coarse string so tightly that severe wounds or mortification frequently occurs.

In China, it is customary to " let out " pain in the head by piercing the eyeball or drum of the ear, often producing thereby blindness and deafness.

Some time ago a conversation was heard between some natives of one of these lands on the advantage of having doctors, and one man related how his wife had been treated for a headache. Several old women took her in hand. They bound a towel about her forehead, placed a brass pot on her head, filled the pot with boiling water, and for about two hours kept up the temperature by ladling out the cooling water and adding boiling water in its place. At the end of the two hours the patient had lost her pain. She was dead.*

Dr. Mackenzie wrote from Tientsin : " I was called to attend a woman in one of the yamens, who was suffering from spasmodic asthma, and found a slave girl beating the back of the chest with a large stick like a rolling-pin, with the idea of giving relief." Necrosis and ulcer from the terrible custom of foot-binding in China is very common. The *British Medical Journal* of Jan. 28, 1899 (p. 231), says : " It not infrequently happens that the flesh becomes putrescent during the process of binding and portions slough off from the sole. Sometimes a toe drops off. . . . Elegance is secured at the cost of months of suffering." The hakims of some nations treat rheumatism by sticking long pins into the patient having tow dipped in oil around the heads of the pins. This is lighted and into the wounds thus caused are inserted " medical nails," composed of corrosive sublimate, arsenic and salt. The profuse discharge saps the strength and sometimes destroys the lives of the patients. Another

---
* *Mercy and Truth*, p. 75, Vol. I., 1897.

1ent of rheumatism in the ankles is that of
he back of the heel, scraping away the mus-
down to the bone, filling the cavity with
:r and then stitching up the skin. Gangrene
; an infrequent sequel to such procedure.

l by medical missionaries in China that oc-
1ative physician finding himself unable to
1se of illness of a parent, will order a soup
? flesh cut from the arm of a son or daugh-
:l for us to realize what must be the pain in-
1 an operation, conducted without an anæs-
he roughest and most pitiless manner.

1 from fever, the sufferer in Northern India
be possessed by a demon, and is put in an
:hained hand and foot to a stone block.

he approach of a small-pox epidemic pro-
ed fear which is met by terribly summary
:xtinction by burning the patients alive,
1em over the edge of rapid torrents, or by
:l more painful process of starvation on a
to which they have been carried. " It is
/ork of the missionary physician to over-
1rbarous systems of medical treatment . . .
1te for them the scientific methods, the skill
es of . . . Western Medicine. . . .
1l sisters is the special honor given to en-
:ic Bastilles of the East with healing and
1ake an end by their skilled and beneficent
? barbarous practices of native midwifery,
1y remediable sufferings of their own sex."
ld seek to measure the power of Christian-
l compare the treatment of the sick before
Christ came and where to-day He is
:tlc not known, with that of countries
where His influence has been felt for
generations. We would commend
s subject to any who wish for a new line of
ich will assuredly strengthen their faith in,
1e office of, the principles brought into the
the love-manifestation of God in His

We would not seem to claim that institutions for treatment of the sick were unknown till the advent of Christianity. Far from it. Notably in India, during the
Buddhist ascendency, about 300 B. C., hospitals were
founded. In that country, as well as in Arabia, Egypt,
Greece and Rome, there was constant association of the
healing art with religious functions. But with a few
notable exceptions their methods were a strange medley
of superstitions and incantations, with but little admix-
ture of rational treatment. And in the best examples of
history we see but a faint foreshadowing of pure altruism
and sacrifice for others, which finds so exalted a place in
Christian Medicine.

"Did Athens with three-fourths, and Rome with
three-fifths, of her population in slavery build hospitals
for the sick, the lame, the blind, the insane, the leper?
Did these humanitarian feelings and customs of benevolence arise in India or China or Japan, with their highly
praised, elaborate system of morals? Among Pagan nations there has been high culture, art and eloquence, but
little humanity. Greece and Rome had shrines for num-
berless divinities, forty theatres for amusement, thousands
of perfumery stores, but no shrine for brotherly love, no
almshouse for the poor. Millions of money were expended on convivial feasts, but nothing for orphans or for
homes for widows. 'In all my classical reading,' says
Professor Packard, 'I have never met with the idea of
an infirmary, or hospital, except for sick cats (a sacred
animal) in Egypt.' "*

Dr. Döllinger says : "Among the millionaires of Rome
there was not one who founded a hospice for the poor or a
hospital for the sick."

"The sympathies of the heathen have never extended
beyond the class, or at widest the nation; but those of
Christianity are as wide as the human race. Christianity
alone has established hospitals for an alien race on the
simple ground of a common human brotherhood."†

Christianity was but in its early centuries when Fabiola, a Roman lady of ancient and noble lineage, founded

---

*"The Growth of the Kingdom of God." Sidney Gulick. p. 265.
†"Life of Peter Parker, M.D." 1896. p. 345.

the first famous Christian hospital. This hospital was situated some distance from the city, in a healthy location. Its fame, we are told, spread throughout the Roman Empire " from the Egyptians and Parthians to the cities of Britain." Fabiola sold her very large patrimony and founded a convalescent home in connection with the hospital. " She constituted herself a nurse, the first of her order, and was in the habit of bearing the sick about, and of bathing their sores on which others would not look. No less generous of her person than of her purse, she braved discomfort that would have discouraged others and seemed to feel that in caring for the wounds of her patients she was caring for those of her Saviour. The same devotion is praised also in the case of the Empress Flacilla, who went herself to the hospitals, took care of the sick, prepared their food, tasted their drink, and performed for them all the duties of a menial ; and when they sought to turn her from her purpose, she replied : ' Let the Emperor distribute his gold ; this I will do for them on whose behalf he holds his Empire.' "* It is only on the banks of the stream that flows from the throne of God that there grows the tree whose leaves are for the healing of the nations.

Cruelty to Insane. Look at the treatment of the insane in these lands and compare it with that in Syria, China, Arabia or Persia. In the latter country, " the poor lunatic is chained, his feet fastened in the stocks, is constantly beaten and half starved with the idea that if badly treated the devil will the sooner leave him. And then, as a last resource when the friends have grown tired of even this unkind care of their relative, the lunatic is given freedom in the desert. His hands are tied behind his back and he is led out into the desert and is never heard of again."

We believe we are right in stating that there is not a single asylum for the treatment of the insane by modern principles in the whole of Syria and Persia, though probably before the year has passed there will be one established at Lebanon. Mr. Waldmeier, to whose earnest advocacy, together with that of two eminent asylum

---

* "Hospitals and Asylums of the World," Burdette, Vol. III., p. 34.

physicians, this first asylum will be mainly due, records that the condition of the mentally diseased in Syria defies description. "A young fellow of twenty-three years became insane with acute mania. Of course, he was chained and actually walled up in a cave. Through a hole they used to throw him sometimes a few dried figs and some bread. He became just like a wild beast; his nails grew long like claws, and he used to tear the rats and mice which were in that abode into pieces to satisfy his hunger. . . . He did more that would be unseemly to mention. He was relieved by death at last, having been in this fearful state for four years." Another patient in a different part of Syria was put in iron chains and given in charge of two merciless fellows, who beat him until relieved by death.

"The Muhammedans have a place at Nablous for those who have lost their reason, and this place is called El Khudr, the patron of which is the prophet Elijah, who shows his power in casting out devils from the madjaneen. If there is any Muhammedan who is madjanoon, they bring him to El Khudr at Nablous. There he is put at once into a horrible position; his arms and feet are put around a pillar, and as they are not long enough to meet they are fastened together with chains. In this cruel position the poor sufferer sits naked, day and night, on the ground, deprived of the use of his arms and feet. A little food is given him by the man who has the oversight of the place. Of cleanliness we cannot think here; the filth defies description. A Muhammedan sheikh comes from time to time and reads to the insane portions from the Koran, and implores the prophet Elijah to cast the demon out from the man. Then the sheikh binds amulets around his arms and feet as charms and bleeds him in different parts of the body." In this Bicêtre of the East no Pinel has yet arisen to unchain the maniac and inaugurate more rational lines of treatment.

The writer will never forget a conversation he had one morning on the steps of a hotel in Jerusalem concerning the care of the insane. The proprietor was speaking with the earnestness and conviction of one who himself had come into contact with the terrible lack of proper pro-

care of such cases. A friend in a compara-
ımily had become mentally afflicted and no
could be found for his reception. " Surely,"
" if Christians believed what they say they
vould seek out and care for those who have
e for them." " Care for those who have no
for them "—the words rang through our
.veeks afterward. Was not this exactly the
vhich Christ came? They that are whole
of a physician, but they that are sick.
ier would urge the objection that such work
less for the extension of the Kingdom of
d give a two-fold reply. Firstly, if this is a
)erative duty toward humanity, who of us
gh to deny its religious importance, both as
dience to the laws of the love-life, and as
demonstration of that life before others?
would remind such objectors that many
nity are showing with modern treatment a
) varying from forty to sixty per cent.
be worth while to do this work for the sake
rtion of cases whose recovery will be as-
o, therefore, will come as legitimately into
vangelizing efforts as any other sick or dis-
lands? It is instructive to us to remember
ction the example of Jesus Christ toward
-e mentally unsound in His day.
ot only is there cruelty in these dark places
the earth, but there is abundant evidence
ivilized communities, is indictable criminal
s well as pure cruelty and neglect. " It is not
lygamous households for discarded or un-
es to bribe the midwife to inflict such an
1e favorite wife as shall render her incapa-
· child-bearing." Mrs. Bird-Bishop states
er travels in Asia she was asked no fewer
; for drugs which would take away a favor-
? know that abortion-mongers are by no
1ent in the great cities of Christian lands.
ast they have to pursue their craft secretly,
e pressure of a growingly healthy public

opinion on the matter.   Where there are no licenses required to practice Medicine, where superstition and gross
ignorance combine to allow anything to be done which
is dictated by the priest-physician or meddlesome midwife, where there is no such thing as healthy public opinion, there are the very elements in which the charlatan
can flourish and pursue his abominable, nefarious and
deadly traffic.

The immoral procedures to which thousands of women
are subjected in the name of medicine in these countries
are beyond recital on the printed page or the public plat-
form.   Occasionally the press in our own land rings with
the story of some poor fellow who has degraded his professional knowledge to ruin morally and physically a weak
and ignorant woman.   The conscience of noble womanhood tingles at the thought of such degradation to one of
their sex.

A great American preacher has said that one of the
supremest contributions of Christianity is the gift of a
burning heart to a world out of heart.   The religion of
Jesus is, after all, the jubilee of kindheartedness, the
epiphany of exalted womanhood.   The high position of
women to-day is the product of Christianity.   Shall not,
then, the hearts of Christian women burn within them as
Jesus Himself draws near and interprets to them from
these new scriptures of knowledge the things concerning
Himself?   It is the Master who is suffering in the persons
of those who are sick and in prison and are left uncared
for, untended and unvisited.

Here is far more than mere cruelty or immorality.   It
is touching the secret springs of a nation's life.   It is of
imperial importance.   If the wife and mother be degraded,
love cannot flourish and the home is blasted.   If the home
is blasted the national unit of strength is destroyed and
there is moral decadence.   This is exactly the sight with
which we are confronted in these lands.   Women of America and women of Britain, will you not rise to this opportunity for rescuing not only the women in these countries,
but also, through them, purifying, ennobling and uplifting
the national life and conscience?

The sick and injured of these lands are crushed like

pack-ice between two approaching icebergs. On the one side is disease claiming from them their life; on the other are the hardly less agonizing attempts at treatment. " Quackery is a miasmatic jungle around which the clean vitalizing work of the Gospel stands out wholesomely."

Even when death is approaching, similar **Cruelty to the** cruel practices are persisted in. An aged **Doors of Death.** parent sick and dying is often carried off to a hilltop and left there with a pot of water and a few barley balls, to perish. " In China, when all hope is given up of a patient's recovery, the custom is to dress them at once in grave clothes and to remove them to a board and trestles away from the ordinary bed, so that it shall not be defiled." Their diagnosis of approaching death is none too accurate, so that it often happens that the closing hours or days are spent in terrible discomfort and pain and the end hastened by this shameful neglect. A missionary wrote us recently from North China, saying he had been called in to a case of a man who was dying. The hubbub of wailing and lamentation was so great as to make conversation with the patient almost impossible.*

We would mentally contrast such scenes with those in the home lands when relatives and friends are passing from us to be with Him. Here all is done in those closing hours which love and forethought can devise for the amelioration of pain and the quiet peacefulness of the sick one. There it is noise and din, wailing and mourning, cold and neglect, and utter and hopeless darkness.

" The paths of pain are thine. Go forth
   With patience, trust and hope ;
The sufferings of a sin-sick earth
   Shall give thee ample scope.

---

* " The sick, if homeless, are transported from doorway to doorway, since it is the legal custom to hold a man responsible for the funeral expenses of a stranger dying at his gate. and he is, moreover, exposed to blackmail under such suspicious circumstances. In Korea an instance is recorded in a recent communication from a missionary, in which a sick man was hurriedly transported from village to village for a period of five days, without food, the inhabitants of each village fearing. in case he should die within its precincts, ' that his spirit would remain to haunt them and work them mischief.' " (Christian Missions and Social Progress. Dr. Jas. S. Dennis. Vol. I.)

Beside the unveiled mysteries
  Of life and death go stand,
With guarded lips and reverent eyes,
  And pure of heart and hand.

So shalt thou be with power endowed
  From Him who went about
The Syrian hillsides doing good
  And casting demons out.

That good Physician liveth yet,
  Thy friend and guide to be ;
The Healer by Gennesaret
  Shall walk the rounds with thee."

VALUE OF MEDICAL MISSIONS

" He is a path, if any be misled ;
He is a robe, if any naked be ;
If any chance to hunger, He is bread ;
If any be a bondman, He is free ;
If any he but weak, how strong is He !
To dead men, life He is ; to sick men health,
To blind men sight, and to the needy wealth ;
A pleasure without loss, a treasure without stealth."

" A thing is great partly by its traditions and partly by its opportunities—partly by what it has accomplished and partly by the doors of serviceableness of which it holds the key."

—George Adam Smith.

" A Christian man is the most free lord of all, and subject to none ; a Christian man is the most dutiful servant of all and subject to every one."

—Martin Luther.

"I will follow that system of regimen which, according to my ability and judgment, I consider for the benefit of my patients, and abstain from whatever is deleterious and mischievous. I will give no deadly medicine to anyone if asked, nor suggest any such counsel. . . . With purity and with holiness I will pass my life and practice my art."

—Hippocrates' Oath, from " Genuine Works of Hippocrates," by Frances Adams.

34

III

VALUE OF MEDICAL MISSIONS

The reasons for Medical Missions are by
no means exhausted by the consideration of
the physical needs in heathen lands resulting from ignorance, superstition, cruelty
ractice.

ong argument for the association of physicans
ionary operations might be built up on the sin-
: the requirements of other missionaries and their
or medical aid. Every year a little army sails
istian lands as missionaries. This wave of con-
ife breaks not only on distant shores, but is car-
iland away from many of the resources of mod-
ation. Every missionary represents his coun-
s Church and their reputation in a measure rests
. The responsibility for their health is one of
oment, considered even on the low ground of the
t which the Boards are at for their transporta-
e field.

rilized government sends its agents on an expe-
a difficult climate without adequate medical as-
Modern warfare depends for success as much
ration against fevers as on shot and shell
ful marksmanship. Yet scores of Ameri-
Europeans are in the mission field with their
ar away from any skill in the time of sickness.
realize the value of these lives, when we remem-
rge proportion of missionaries' children who in
me missionaries, one sees in a new light the holy
of being able to prolong their lives by thought-
: and to save them when the ravages of climate
their best to break and shatter their health.

In Turkey some years ago a missionary's child died; a second died; then a third little one was taken. The fourth was ill, and the parents made a desperate effort to reach a doctor in time. They went a long journey, only to hear the verdict "too late" and to turn homeward, bringing back with them their last child to lay beside the other three.

"In the interior of most foreign lands the only medical aid available is that rendered by the missionary doctor. Excepting in the principal seaports of China, Africa and Turkey, in the large cities and cantonment centres of India, and in a few corresponding places in other lands, the only skilled physicians at hand are those possessed by the missions themselves. It is a matter that calls for gratitude to God that the lives of the missionaries—the most valuable commodity of a mission—have frequently been saved, their health preserved and sickness avoided by the timely attendance and advice of the resident missionary physician. It is a matter to be regretted that not infrequently devoted and earnest missionaries eager to preach the Gospel in new and remote districts have prematurely sacrificed their lives or permanently injured their health for the cause, when with a knowledge of Medicine in their own part, or the help of a competent physician, they might have saved them, to the greater good and enlargement of the work they sought to establish."*

Again and again a missionary has to make a journey of hundreds of miles, where traveling is excessively slow, in order to reach some medical mission and consult the physician there on his own behalf or for a wife or child with whom he has had to journey. This is not only a very expensive matter in money, but also dislocates the work of the mission by the enforced and prolonged absence of one or more missionary agents. It is, of course, recognized that in some parts of the field medical missionaries are not required and would be superfluous. But that is not true of vast tracts of unoccupied territory which could best be reached through the association of medical work with that of the ordinary clerical missionary. Ought there not to be a medical missionary

---

* The Medical Mission. W. J. Wanless. p. 58 *et seq.*

within easy access of every considerable mission station for the maintenance of the health of those workers, as well as for his or her own special influence?

Value to the Profession at Home.

The opportunities of practice abroad are far more numerous than at home. Our profession needs the contributions of this immense field of clinical experience. Already workers in mission lands have rendered valuable service in many departments. This has been notably so in such subjects as tropical fevers, tumors, calculi, eye and skin diseases. The enormous number of cases passing annually through the hands of many mission surgeons make their records and generalizations of peculiar importance.

We note that in one hospital in North India during 1897, 1,200 operations were performed on the eye and nearly 100 malignant tumors were removed. We understand that this was the work of two surgeons. It is recorded of Dr. Kerr, of China, one of the oldest medical missionaries, that he has had 700,000 cases which have been aided, that he has performed 40,000 operations and stands second only to Sir William Thompson in the number of times he has operated for calculus—1,300 times.

The gain to the profession at large would have been far greater if medical missionaries had possessed greater leisure. The overworked and undermanned condition of almost every medical mission has made the task of collaboration of experience an excessively difficult one. Yet they stand in these far away outposts of the world in a position where they can render very real service by the records of their experience, which will be of value to their successors on the field and through the profession to governments and to commerce.

Moreover, not only does our profession claim the results of such unique experience, but it needs medical missionaries for its *own* sake.

New temptations are springing up in the spirit of commercialism, overriding and selfish ambition which threaten to rob the profession of Medicine of something which has so illumined it in the past. "The practice of the healing art is an occupation intrinsically dignified. The true physician recognizes in the most abject human being a fellow man and in the most exalted nothing more."

" We claim to constitute or represent a liberal profession and the very idea or essence of a liberal profession, as distinguished from a trade, is that the acquisition of money is not its primary object."

Again and again this nobility has been strenuously maintained. When some feeble attempts were made to obtain a patent for the use of ether or to keep secret the process of etherization, or when within the past few months a patent was sought for the preparation of an antitoxin, the indignation of the profession was aroused. " The money changers were driven from the temple of humanity."

Prof. Geo. H. Wilson was responsible for the statement many years ago that " the gratuitous professional services of medical men far exceed in number and weight the gratuitous professional services of ministers of all Churches or denominations."

Our great profession in every age has had the reputation of nobility and self-sacrifice. This is one of our most precious heritages. We can conceive of few things which will so maintain this high repute and ennoble and glorify its beneficent character as the going forth from the midst of it of a band of men and women to surrender their talents for those who are in physical and spiritual destitution. As a great surgeon* said, " We ask you to honor the profession by helping it to honor and adorn itself, by helping it to write on the bells of the horses, ' Holiness unto the Lord,' by helping it to be instrumental in saving the souls as well as the bodies of men, by helping it to place in its coronet new jewels of greatest value and brightest lustre, by helping it to twine in its garland a new wreath from the ever-green and ever-growing plant of renown." In thus honoring the profession we shall honor the profession's Head, the Lord Healer, God, who became man, and bore our sicknesses and carried our sorrows.

All we have we owe to God. " Ought " is just

---
* Late Dr. Miller, Professor of Surgery, Edinburgh University.

The Need to GOD. the old Anglo-Saxon for "owe." Talent is a debt of obligation. He is no longer on earth as man, but His command still endures, " Go . . . heal . . . preach." The withdrawal of miraculous cures is no better reason for ceasing the work of healing which He began than is the disappearance of miraculous gifts of tongues a reason for ceasing to study language in order to preach the Gospel of the Kingdom of Heaven.

God is no longer manifested in human form, going in and out among our sick ones. The hand of Christ is no longer laid on the fevered brow; it is for your hand to do that now and to reduce the fever by all the means within your power. His touch of the sightless eyeballs does not to-day restore vision. He has commissioned you to do that with your cataract needle and to be a light to the inly blind, showing forth the Father that He may be glorified in your good works. The summer evenings when the sick could be gathered at the door for the Master to heal have sped away from the world's Capernaums; He is seeking for representatives to-day who shall go in Christ's stead and do His healing work, beseeching men to be reconciled to Him. His wondrous works were tokens of superior knowledge and power. He has given the key of knowledge and power to us to acquire by diligent study. Is not the power with which He entrusts us even greater than that of the early disciples whose work was but for a few years and was local and limited in its operation?

GOD NEEDS YOU. Eighteen hundred years ago He said, " Go ye into all the world and preach the Gospel o the whole creation . . . and these signs shall follow . . . they shall lay their hands on the sick and hey shall recover."

To-day, half the world has never heard those good idings. He has given to medical men a talent of singuar power for proclaiming that message. What are we loing with it?

esults of Medical Missions—as a Pioneer Agent. The benefits of Medical Missions as a pioneer agency have proved themselves so great as to form an argument for the immediate and widespread increase of this method of work. Time and again

doors fast closed against the ordinary missionary have
been gladly opened to the healer-preacher. Twice had
the Church Missionary Society tried to enter Kashmir;
and twice had they failed.   Then Elmslie was sent
as a Medical Missionary.   His splendid services as a
surgeon gradually broke down prejudices and now for
many years there has been a most successful missionary
station in that province.

A few years ago Dr. MacKinnon was trying to secure
ground for a hospital in Damascus.   The fanatical Moslem population of the city opposed his claims.   Just at
this time " a judge in one of the law courts of Damascus
came in hot haste to the house of Dr. MacKinnon and be-
sought him to rush off at once to the abode of the Chief
Cadi.   ' What is wrong?' said the English hakim. ' Have
pity and come at once! ' was the eager response; ' The Cadi's little boy, so dearly loved, is very, very ill.'   The doctor went and was promptly shown in.   The inmates were
in great alarm; dread and disquietude were everywhere
apparent.   Ushered into the sick chamber, the English hakim saw a child of three years, livid and well nigh pulse-
less. A glance at the child, a glance around and the diagnosis is made—opium poisoning.   Then and there began a
struggle with death.   For full two hours he fought and
wrought, stimulating the dying boy and keeping up constant artificial respiration.   A hard and anxious fight
it was, but in the end death was routed.   Slowly the flick-
ering signs of life grew stronger and steadier, until at
last anxiety began to lose itself in gratitude and in praise
to God.   With words of heartfelt thanks the powerful
Cadi embraced the foreigner, declaring that through life
he is his debtor."   The result of all this was that the
Cadi, who was chief presiding officer of the court, began to display a new interest in the pending lawsuit, and
did his best to push the case rapidly through and see that
justice was done to the missionary.   The tide of feeling
among the people quite turned in favor of the doctor, and
they paid him the unusual compliment of rising from
their seats the next time he entered the law court.

Dr. Nevius says that he was at one time trying to establish a station in an interior city of China and was find-

ing great difficulty because of the prejudice and superstition of the people. One day when speaking to a crowd a soldier forced his way up and addressed him very respectfully, showing a deep scar on his cheek. He said that he had been severely wounded in battle and that in the hospital in Shanghai Dr. Lockhart had dressed and healed his wounds. Incidents like that do more to disarm suspicion of the motives of missionary work than any other thing.

At the risk of repeating an old story we quote the incident of Kenneth Mackenzie's pioneering work in one of the large Chinese cities.* " Tien-tsin furnishes a romance in the history of medical missions. When Dr. J. Kenneth Mackenzie reached this city in March, 1879, everything looked dark for the medical mission. While at prayer with the native converts, a member of the English Legation learned that the wife of the Viceroy was seriously ill, the doctors having wholly despaired of her case. The Englishman entering an earnest plea for the foreign doctors, the Viceroy committed his wife's case to the care of Dr. Mackenzie, who was speedily summoned to the vice-regal palace, and in a few weeks Lady Li was quite well. Her treatment was followed by successful surgical operations in the presence of the Viceroy. The court was stirred and great public interest excited. The Viceroy agreed to pay the current expenses of both a hospital and dispensary when erected. In a short time a building was completed with wards for sixty patients, the Chinese themselves contributing the sum of $10,000."

† " If you will try and realize the conditions of an Eastern city," writes the Doctor, " you will quickly understand that when a great potentate takes you by the hand the land is all before you. So we found that in our daily visits to our noble patient our steps were thronged with eager suppliants, who, hearing that the Viceroy's wife was undergoing medical treatment, sought for relief from the same source. You know how a story often grows as it spreads, and so this case of cure was being magnified into a miracle of healing. A Chinese official residence is

---

* Encyclopedia of Missions. 1891. Vol. II., p. 52.
† Biography J. K. Mackenzie, p. 180.

composed of numerous quadrangles, one behind the other, with buildings and gateways surrounding each. To reach the family apartments we had to pass through these numerous courts and here we were beset with patients from the crowds assembled outside the gates, and the friends of soldiers, doorkeepers, secretaries and attendants who had succeeded in gaining an entrance. The poor also besieged us as we entered and left the yamen. It was truly a strange gathering we found daily collected round the outer gates—the halt, the blind and the deaf were all there waiting to be healed; indeed, the whole city seemed to be moved. High officials sought introductions to us through the Viceroy himself."

During Lady Li's illness, Miss L. H. Howard, M. D., an American missionary, was installed in a suite of rooms in the official residence adjoining her ladyship's apartments. It is inconceivable that any other form of missionary agency could have produced such an impression in so short a time as to make these procedures possible.

The Hon. John W. Foster, ex-Secretary of State, says: "A special feature in the mission work of the world, to which great enlargement has been given in late years, is the Medical Missionary. We found that in China, where the science of surgery is almost unknown, they were proving a most helpful adjunct of the work, a door of access to the people not otherwise reached, a ready means of overcoming prejudice and opposition. I am pleased to bear hearty testimony to the scientific attainments and the Christian zeal of the male and female workers in this department and to commend the field as one which can never be overcrowded by the Church at home."

Several years ago, Dr. Valentine settled down at work as a medical missionary in an Indian city. God laid His strong hand upon him in a serious illness—a hand which has so often been laid upon His servants to lead them forth into a larger life and fuller, more influential service. Valentine had been recommended to go to the great snowy Himalayas for change and rest. Mountains, especially snow-clad ones, are Nature's rejuvenators, even in expectation and in memory. On his way he passed through Jeypore and paid a formal call on the Maharajah. " The

Maharajah told him that his wife, the Maharanee, was very ill, and that the native physicians had given her up. Dr. Valentine said that he would be glad to see her and do what he could for her. The way was opened up. The Maharajah was pleased and arranged, difficult as it is to gain access to the women there, that Dr. Valentine should visit the Ranee. . . . The result was that through God's blessing upon Dr. Valentine's treatment the Maharanee was restored to health. The Maharajah said, 'What can I do for you?' He replied, Let me preach the Gospel here.' The Maharajah said, If you will stay here and be my private physician, I shall be glad.' Dr. Valentine rejoined, ' But I am a missionary of the Gospel.' (No missionary had previously been allowed to settle in Jeypore, that great stronghold of idolatry, perhaps one of the greatest strongholds in Northern India.) The Maharajah asked, ' But you will be my private physician, will you not?' He replied, ' Yes, but only upon one condition, that you will allow me to preach the Gospel from one end of the province to the other without let or hindrance.' The Maharajah agreed and Dr. Valentine remained at Jeypore for fourteen years."

"The Medical Missionary has often been able to penetrate out-of-the-way places, places where religious opposition has been most severe and race barriers most formidable, districts where the severity of the climate has made it unsafe for any but the medical missionary to enter. With his healing mission as his defense, and the Word of God as his weapon, the medical missionary has been able to safely traverse tracts of country never before trod by Christian feet. In districts once visited his return is eagerly looked for. And in the train of his pioneering labors other forms of mission work beside his own have been duly inaugurated. For his sake other missionaries are not only tolerated, but frequently welcomed. The physician's presence has not only saved the precious lives of other missionaries, but has often made the continuance of a station possible, when, otherwise, abandonment would have been inevitable. . . . It is, moreover, a fact that not only have individuals been approached, homes entered, stations occupied and districts prepared by the medical missionary which apparently could not have been effected by any other class of workers, but whole countries have been opened up to the Gospel by the elemental labors of missionary physicians."*

It has been said that " China was opened to the Gospel at the point of the lancet " by Dr. Peter Parker. Dr. Allen, an American medical missionary, was the first Protestant foreigner to reside permanently in Korea. He was ultimately put in charge of a hospital built for him by the King of Korea, and later he was one of a Korean Embassy to the United States Government at Washington.

Formosa was opened up largely by the work of medical missionaries. Dr. G. L. Mackay, of the Canadian Presbyterian Mission, was the pioneer missionary to North Formosa, and the first to build a hospital there. At the outset he had almost to compel his patients to come to him. During fourteen years of service he extracted 21,000 teeth in his hospital and on tours, and by this simple operation he has won his way to the hearts of thousands of people.

Siam is another illustration of a country opened up to mission work largely through the influence of the missionary physicians, Drs. Gützlaff, Bradley and House being the pioneers. In Japan, during the inception of missionary work, fields outside of the open ports were opened and held by the establishment of dispensaries by medical missionaries. At the centres where medical work was carried on, it broke down the prejudices and opposition of religious teaching and opened the way for general evangelical work.

Similarly in the Turkish Empire, Persia, Arabia, and throughout the length and breadth of the great Dark Continent of Africa have medical missionaries been used of God in preparing the way for the coming of His Kingdom. There are certain fields of missionary endeavor where Medical Missions appear destined to exert a peculiarly powerful influence. This would seem to be especially true in Muhammedan countries. The comparative neglect of the strongholds of Islam has been one of the darkest shadows resting upon missionary polity. The

*The Medical Mission. W. J. Wanless. Chap. VI., p. 47.

lifficulties of such work are enormous. Opposition has
)een fierce; ignorance and fanatical bigotry have been
:ncountered in their most belligerent forms. The evan-
;elization of Muhammedan people has been called the
;ibraltar of Heathendom, the impregnable rock against
vhich Christianity has seemed to make little progress.
\ny plan of operations professing to be specially adapted
o overthrow these great and allied forces deserves most
:arnest consideration. Medical Missions claim to constitute
uch a plan. At Busrah, Arabia, Dr. Worrell treated
learly 1,000 Moslems during 1897, and by this means the
;ospel was proclaimed to hundreds, scarcely one of whom,
)ut for the medical work, would have come within sound
)f the good tidings of salvation.

Similar testimony comes from Ispahan, Persia, West
\frica, Egypt, Palestine, and Kashmir. " No student of
Medical Missions will challenge the statement that Med-
cal Missions are the most important manifestation at the
)resent time in the whole world of the practical spirit of
Christianity." It is this essentially practical character
vhich appeals to the feelings of those whose hearts are
:ase-hardened against the impact of doctrine. It is the
:esame which opens the heart when the keys of persua-
ion, argument, invitation and education have failed to
nove the bolt. The medical missionary has not to go out
nd seek the indifferent. They come to him of their own
iccord; perhaps at first it is but for the material bene-
ts which he can confer upon them, but this affords him
 splendid theatre of demonstrating Christianity in action,
vhich, followed up by teaching, rapidly breaks down
)igotry and makes the patient realize in the physician a
ellow man who has a higher, deeper and sweeter motive
n life than any to which his creed has given him access.

esults of, Medical It has been stated that Dr. Mackenzie, of
Issions — Spiritu- Tien-tsin, was made instrumental in
ly Numerous and bringing more souls to Christ in one year
Par-reaching. than all the other members of the mission
put together. We would not, however,
take the reputation of Medical Missions on any such sta-
istical ratio of conversions compared with those due to
)ther forms of work. If the results were tabulated, it

would probably be found that Medical Missions were able
to show a smaller proportion of conversions than other
lines of missionary activity. When one remembers how
many seemed to come to Christ, seeking only that their
lameness might be healed, or their leprosy cleansed, and
caring little or nothing for His invitation, " Take My
yoke upon you and learn of Me," we are not surprised if
the same be true with His followers.

> "Yet it was well, and Thou hast said in season,
>   ' As is the Master shall the servant be.'
> Let me not subtly slide into the treason
>   Seeking an honor which they gave not Thee."

We believe that if the results were but one-tenth of
what they are, they would still be worth having because
the prosecution of such work is a magnificent object-les-
son. Many of these children, standing in shadow, in spiritual intelligence, will appreciate better the spectacular
tableaux vivantes of Christian love than a closely reasoned
thesis on the subject.

But the results of medical evangelism are by no
means small. They are both numerous and far-reaching.
The Bishop of Victoria, Hong Kong, who has been connected with the diocese twenty-two years, says, " I have
known convert after convert in our hospital at Ningpo,
and I can certainly point most distinctly to three churches
which have been born in it." The first convert of that
hospital was an opium smoker, who came to be cured. He
asked that an evangelist might be sent to his own home in
a distant city. One was sent and two years later thirty-
seven converts were baptized through the work of the
hospital patient and the native preacher. Now there is
a strong church of 700 baptized believers.

One of the medical missionaries of the London Mission at Amoy, China, states that 1,200 to 1,400 towns and
villages are yearly represented at the hospital. As a
result of the cure of one man seventeen years ago, no less
than seven Christian congregations have been formed,
with a membership of from thirty to one hundred in each.
Dr. Gillison told the author of seven men coming to his
hospital at Hankow from a distance of 320 miles. He
operated for cataract on the eye of one man and restored

the sight. He said he would do the same for the other eye in three months' time. Gillison forgot about the case, but three months after the man returned with forty-seven others!

In reply to inquiries in a Chinese city, one well-known worker says: " Nearly all admitted to the church in this city have been brought in through the hospital." Another estimates that " one-third of the membership is the result of the influence of hospital work." Another writes, " The majority of those who have been admitted here to our church were from the hospital." A writer in the *Church Missionary Intelligencer* says: " I will mention one thing that I learned in talking with the American missionaries. They told me—several, if not all of them—that they scarcely ever met with a person interested in Christianity, or a Christian inquirer, in the villages within a radius of 150 miles from Hang-chow who had not been brought to be interested and to inquire through the means . . . of . . . teaching in hospital." The twenty-second annual report of the Mission to Lepers in India and the East mentions that more than 200 lepers had confessed Christ. There are now over 1,000 professing Christians in these leper asylums.

In China a missionary physician successfully operated on the eyes of a parent and her two daughters. The mother had never gazed into the faces of her children before, and her delight and gratitude knew no bounds. The light shone in further and deeper than mere visual perception and revealed to her and her daughters the sight of the Lord Jesus standing over them as the One Who had died to save and redeem. Father and mother and both girls were converted and through their influence a successful little church of a hundred persons now meets for worship in their village.

And the influence of Medical Missions is far-reaching in more than a geographical sense. " Now I hold," wrote a Chinese missionary, " that of the thirty thousand who have passed through our wards and whose homes are scattered over an area three or four times larger than England, everyone may be taken as a centre of influence more or less favorable to Western thought and Western men,

and so to the messengers of Christ, and thus by the work
done at our . . . hospital we are preparing the way
for future conversions on a pentecostal scale."

Many definite spiritual results must ever be unknown.
This is naturally the case when the attraction of medical
aid draws patients from far-away places to which they
return when cured, and are often lost to subsequent ob-
servation. The germinating power of this seed, sown in
uncongenial soil away from Christian help and sympathy,
is constantly filling those on the field with praise.

Some years ago a mandarin who had lost his nose presented himself before a medical missionary. He had
heard of the high repute of the foreign physician and he
wanted to test it by getting him to make him a new nose.
Other surgeons had been asked, but all were too busy
with more important duties. At length he reached this
hospital, 1,000 miles from home. The doctor took him in
for three months and then he went away with what he
came for—a new nose. " It was not a very handsome
one," says the doctor, " but was a nose, made of his own
flesh and blood. He said I had made him a foreigner's
nose instead of a Chinaman's, but he was so proud of it,
nevertheless, that he carried a little mirror in his sleeve,
and was continually looking at this new facial ornament.
This gentleman took away from our hospital also something which he did not come for—a more or less extensive
knowledge of the Gospel . . . and while in the hospital had read the New Testament through and through.
But he read it only that he might argue against it, and
when he left us was so bitterly opposed to Christianity
that I put him down in my notebook as ' a surgical success, but an evangelical failure.' That entry I must now
confess was a record of lack of faith in me. I ought to
have known that so much Gospel truth was not likely to
lie dormant in that man's heart, and it did not. Last year
the news reached me that in his distant home that gentleman had gone to the missionary, professed his faith in
Jesus and had been received by baptism into the Christian
Church." Doubtless, in scores and hundreds of villages
in India, China and elsewhere there are similar cases.
Surely, surely, the results of Medical Missions are spiritu-
ally numerous and far-reaching!

INFLUENCE OF MEDICAL MISSIONS

" Religion has ever been the saving force in human history. How otherwise can we explain the moral helplessness and social decay of humanity, as a universal rule, up to the present hour, wherever the spiritual inspiration and the ethical force of religion have been absent? Left to itself, society seems to be self-destructive and to have no remedy within its own resources."

—*James S. Dennis, D.D.*

" Sacrifice is the language of love. Those who do not sacrifice are like men living on the top of gold mines, or sailing across beds of pearl oysters, unconscious of the riches within their very reach. It is no sacrifice to give a cup of cold water when a cup of something better is within reach."

—*War Cry.*

" I thought these men will carry hence
Promptings their former life above,
And something of a finer reverence
For beauty, truth and love."

—*James Russell Lowell.*

" In effecting any radical changes of this kind, doubtless there would be great inconvenience and loss incurred by al' the originators of the movement. That which can be done with perfect convenience and without loss is not always the thing that most needs to be done, or which we are imperatively required to do."

—*John Ruskin.*

IV

INFLUENCE OF MEDICAL MISSIONS

Results Abide in Memory and Win Gratitude. The work of medical missionaries not only touches the tenderest side of man, but they impress his memory and abide in his thoughts more persistently than words which he hears. The kindly forethought and patient attention of some friend to us when we were ill cannot be effaced from the pages of remembrance even when all his words have been forgotten.

Sickness is a Valley of Humiliation; there is little sublimity in the sick-room; it is suggestive of helplessness. Men feel when prostrated by illness much like Napoleon returning baffled from Moscow—"God Almighty has been too much for me." The stronger and more active the life has been in the past in succoring others, the more keenly does it feel the humiliation of being served. Much of this feeling is a healthy manifestation of dislike for all that is frail and maimed and decrepit. In nature we see this strong bias acting beneficially in the evolution of the race, by placing an embargo upon all that is weak and unfitted for life's strain and struggle. One of the wonders of Christianity has been the transformation of this weakness into might of character; this humiliation of body into spiritual triumph.

The sickly sentimentality of a generation ago, which made it appear that beauty of soul was only attained through weakness of body, and that made all good children die young after protracted illnesses, was but a parasite and parody foisted upon the true parable of pain. Character, robust, resourceful and ready for active service, is still formed in the rough battleground of life, where strength meets strength and grapples for the victory. But the service Christianity has rendered is to show that there are other schools of character, and that the product of such teaching as pain and sickness may be no less noble and forceful in uplifting power than that produced in the roar of the busy mart or amid the rattle of shot and shell.

The Christian faith, therefore, has a message of courage and hope to bring to the sick-bed and the very nature of illness makes the sufferer especially ready to receive it. Life wears a busy aspect to the poor of these countries where so little is earned by such great labor. Many feel that they have not time to look into the matter of this foreigner's religion; they are not specially interested in it. To others of official class or high birth, the thought of social degradation is enough to keep them from close inquiry. Even if they listen in a bazar or a preaching hall, enough is not gleaned to enable them to fully understand the purport of the message. But overtaken by accident or sickness, either class may be ready then to surrender prejudices for the sake of the physical benefits which they know the foreign doctor can bestow. Lying week after week in hospital, knowledge of the doctrine deepens and gratitude awakes. This gratitude is often most touching and is exhibited years after the patient has left hospital.

Dr. Douthwaite, of Chefoo, relates that when leaving the city the general in command, with his officers, came with a regiment of soldiers and lined up before the hospital. On going out to them they dropped on their knees and stayed there while one of their number addressed the doctor, thanking him for his services. The Emperor of China showed his appreciation of the medical missionaries' work during the recent war by conferring on several of them the Order of the Double Dragon.

" The father, whose only child, a beautiful daughter, had a tumor of seven pounds weight removed from her back, after she was discharged well, returned with a scroll bearing a poetical inscription to the physician to this effect: 'A grievous disease had entwined itself around my little daughter; I had gone in various directions, seeking for physicians of distinction, and had expended much money upon them in vain. When I heard of the foreign physician in the provincial city, I took my little daughter by the hand, and repaired to his residence with the speed of a courser. He received and treated my daughter, removing the flaw from the gem, and now she is a perfect pearl again."

Often a patient returns in gratitude to thank the mission surgeon and has to be restrained from falling down and worshipping him. Some of these expressions of thanks, mingled as they are with heathenish ideas, are strong evidences of the influence of missionary medicine.

A woman had come to a mission hospital for cataract. Not long after the operation had been performed, she was seen kneeling with bare knees upon a number of date stones on a brick bed. " Does it not pain you? " she was asked. " Yes," was the reply, " and that is why I am doing it. Since I came to this hospital you have tried to open my eyes, but you have also opened my heart. I have learned of Jesus' love for me. I am poor and aged and can do nothing for Him. Because He has suffered such infinite pain for my sake, I thought to myself I would suffer a little for Him." It was the idea of one just emerging from heathenism, but had insight into the demands made upon her by so great love.

" On one of my recent boat journeys," writes a missionary, " I put in about dusk at the market town of Hwang-sz-Kang, and I had no sooner finished preaching on shore than a man rushed after me on to the boat, with hands full of peaches, which he pressed me to accept. I told him I was not aware that I had done anything to warrant my taking them, but he would hear of no refusal. ' You are from Hankow, are you not? ' ' Yes,' I replied. ' Well, you will probably not remember me, but a few years ago I went up to your hospital there, very ill indeed, and had it not been for Dr. Mackenzie I certainly should not have lived. And not only so, but when all my money was exhausted, he supported me for a whole month and both he and the native assistants treated me with so much kindness that, when I saw you here, knowing as I did that you must be connected with the mission, I thought the least that I could do was to give you some slight acknowledgment of the kindness shown me at Hankow. I am but a poor man, a huckster, and in a very small way, but I shall be only too glad if you will accept these peaches.' And feeling hardly satisfied with this expression of grati-

tude, though a very poor man, he brought later in the
evening a further present of peaches and sweetmeats, to
show how grateful he was for the kindness he had received." We think that the perfume of that fruit must
have been exceeding fragrant and the taste very sweet to
the missionary. When some heaven-born artist

" Shall draw the thing as he sees it
For the God of Things As They Are."

this will be one of the delicate miniatures of loving life
to hang beside the picture of the woman with the alabaster
box. That canvas, like the other, will hold high place in
the gallery of the House Beautiful.

The Chinese used to say of Dr. Fred. Roberts that
they never saw any one so like the Lord Jesus. " If we
want," said Dr. Arthur Lankester, " to write the teaching
of our Lord Jesus Christ in very big letters so that those
who cannot read theology and do not understand science
or philosophy can read it very easily, the best way of doing it, whether it be for an individual, a village, a town, a
district, or a nation, is to start medical aid for the poor."

We may take the Bible to a heathen and he may burn
it or throw it aside. Civilization and education may only
turn him from heathenism into an infidel or materialist.
It may be hard to convince him that you are not preaching for the sake of a salary. But let that man come to
you in bodily distress and be relieved and cured, and he
will learn to love you and be grateful and that is often but
the first step to loving the Saviour Who commissioned you
in this work.

The return of the one leper must have rejoiced the
Master's heart, when, depressed by the heedless ingrati-
tude of the other nine who left Him unthanked for the
work He had wrought. Similar gratitude was recently
expressed by some like afflicted ones in the following
touching words:* " To Our Most Honorable Friends and
Supporters: We, the men and women of the Leper Asylum at Purulia, send you a thousand thanks. We are
well in body so far as may be expected, though some of us
suffer great bodily pains, which have been mitigated, how-

* The Double Cross and Medical Missionary Record, April, 1896. p. 77.

ever, by the kindness you have shown us so continually.
We have now good houses to dwell in, tanks to bathe and
wash in, wells for giving us drinking water, and a doctor
and medicines to heal our ulcers. We have teachers and
pastors who instruct, guide and comfort us. All these
advantages we owe, next to God, to you, our benefactors
and friends. Our nearest relatives have abandoned and
forsaken us, and there is no place left for us on earth
where we could rest and stay without molestation. People seeing us from a distance, shouted, ' Begone! Begone!' Ah, that was hard!" We wonder how many of
ourselves in like condition would be in such a grateful
mood as these lepers. We are reminded of what we think
was a sentence in one of Charles Lamb's letters in which
he thus concludes in substance: " I am just recovering
from pneumonia, and am suffering a good deal with rheumatism and asthma, and have gout; otherwise, I am very
well!"

The Broader Influence of Medical Missions. The bye-products of some mines have become as valuable as the very ore for which the mines were opened. The results of Medical Missions, unplanned and quite unpremeditated, have astonished many who have no interest in the extension of the Kingdom of God, as such. Though the salvation of souls must and shall ever be the cap sheaf and the keystone of Medical Missions, yet these sub-influences are not thereby ruled out of court as unimportant. " In the nature of the case," said Sir William Acland, " Medicine has relation to every individual of the human race in whatever climate, in whatever state of social organization or disorganization; of whatever religion; whether in peace or at war." Missionary Medicine has not exhausted its influence when it has healed the sick one and brought him to know the Christ Who for us men came down to die and Who ever liveth to make intercession. It reaches round and exerts its power on a larger world than that gathered in the hospital waiting room. It pioneers education, it stimulates scientific methods; it inculcates sanitary principles and introduces plague precautions and deals with epidemics. Again and again it becomes of political importance; its weight is

thrown on the side of benevolent undertakings; while all
the time it is raising in estimation the value of human life
and the sacredness of womanhood. These are stars of
the first magnitude, which shine brightly in the firma-
ment of Christian Sociology.

Medical Mission work destroys caste. In the waiting
room of a dispensary may often be seen sitting side by
side the Brahmin, Sudra and Shanar, the Pulayer and Pariah, the devil worshipper, the worshipper of Siva, the
Muhammedan, the Roman Catholic and Protestant, both
men and women of all castes and creeds.

A year or two ago *The Independent* gave an account
of a concert successfully organized by the United States
Minister at Teheran for the benefit of the Presbyterian
Medical Mission in that city. The support accorded it
was an interesting testimony of the way such a mission
appeals to wider humanity. The Diplomatic Corps and a
large number of Persian officials gave their hearty support, and when a subscription list was started it was
headed by the Prime Minister and was contributed to by
every Persian official at the capital as well as the entire
European colony, including Russians and Turks. The
concert was so successful that the Shah himself requested
it to be repeated at the palace and personally received his
guests.

A brilliant writer in the *Daily Telegraph* says: " I
have always acted on the theory that the persons who
know most of the social conditions of any people are the
doctors and the clergy. The one class see the shadier
and the other the brighter side of humanity, but both
go down to the depths. . . . Above all is it the case
where you have medico and parson combined. . . .
There may be better ways of promoting humanity and civilization; if so, one would like to see them at work. . . .
It may be allowed to count in our estimate that once a
week a few hundred thousands of these people are with-
drawn from Sundayless, unresting toil; that they are
taught a higher morality and a nobler theology; that a
ray of brightness now and then is thrown over their lot,
and lives no longer demon-haunted are made happier. At

* *Daily Telegraph*, London, England, July 25, 1898.

any rate, it is safe to say that without the Christian missions there would not exist one single hospital throughout the length and breadth of China.   That, at least, may pass for something."

Many will enthusiastically admit the value of medical work, altogether apart from its religious motive and purpose.   Dr. Coltman relates that when coming across the Pacific he was conversing with a fellow-passenger who professed to be an atheist.   " Well, I can see the good of medical work among the Chinese or any other race who have no scientific treatment of disease. It is humanitarian, and as such I would subscribe to it."

It was this humanitarian spirit in women medical missionaries which helped to create sentiment in India leading to the modification of the marriage laws.   " Such revelations of inhumanity connected with child marriages were brought to light that one of the physicians connected with the Methodist Church drew up a petition which was signed by fifty-five women physicians and presented to the Government, pleading that the marriageable age of girls be raised to fourteen years.   While the Government was flooded with petitions and memorials from native Christians, Hindu women and missionaries, it is stated that nearly all the speakers in the Legislative Council referred to the facts presented in this memorial."   Dr. James Martineau says: " There is not a secular reform in the whole development of modern civilization, which, if it is more than mechanical, has not drawn its inspiration from a religious principle.   Infirmaries for the body have sprung out of duty for the soul; schools for the letter, that free way may be opened for the spirit; sanitary laws, that the diviner elements in human nature may not become hopeless from their foul environment."

Incentive to Higher Education. Many hospitals and dispensaries are training colleges for theoretical and practical instruction in Western medicine.

Thus an opportunity is afforded of bringing the brightest native Christians into a sphere of influence for benefiting future generations.   The work that has been done in these directions is astonishing to any who have acquaintance with the full curriculum and stringent requirements set forth by the missionary teachers.

The plan adopted in most cases is to take in a number of young men at a time for a four or five years' curriculum and to receive no others till their course is completed. This makes it possible for the busy missionary physicians to take up with all the students at once the subjects requisite for the first year ; then to pass to second year subjects, and so on.   Dr. Dugald Christie, of Moukden, Manchuria, began such work single handed with six students for a five years' course, and testifies that these young men have given great satisfaction and promise to become useful workers in the Master's vineyard.   Similar work was carried out in Madagascar a few years ago.   More than one regular college now exists in India for giving like instruction in medicine as a preparation for missionary service.

The course in Beirut Medical School is on a regularly graded system.   It lasts four years.   A preliminary examination in English is required.   The course is very thorough and has reacted on the whole system of medical education in the land and advanced the standard of medical learning.   Dr. Valentine, of India, has been enabled to originate several institutions for the educational improvement of the people, such as a school of art, a library, philosophical institute, museum, as well as examining in government schools and publishing much literature.   Before the first woman missionary physician had left America for India, Dr. Humphrey had begun training a few young women in Medicine.   Now there is a well equipped School of Medicine for native Christian women there.

An Uplifting Power to Womanhood. " Medical work has been a spur to the higher education of women.   It has given woman a higher ideal of life, for every one treated in a hospital learns something of cleanliness and care of the sick, and carries away a treasure of new ideas which cannot fail to bring comfort and health to cheerless homes."

The fact that attention is paid to suffering women by medical missionaries is already changing the prevalent ideas as to the inferiority and worthlessness of their lives.

The seeds are thus being sown for a new harvest of chivalry and reverence toward womankind. The position which medical work holds can hardly be better stated than by the words of a high caste Hindu, who when asked as to the method most likely to convert their people, answered: " We do not fear the usual method of mission work, such as the school, printing-presses and bazar preaching, but we do fear your lady zenana worker, and we dread your lady doctors; they enter our homes, win the hearts of our women, threatening the foundation of our religion." The sociological significance of the single fact that Medical Missions raises the value of human life and elevates the position of women in society can hardly be overestimated. These two moral conceptions alone, enforced by Christian practice, are sufficient to transform the whole social fabric of non-Christian lands.

Contributions to Science. Scientific Medicine has had its traditions maintained by the work done by medical missionaries. These labors have been another factor of sociological importance. *Rev. W. A. P. Martin, President of the Imperial University in Peking, said that it was not easy to estimate the value of the books prepared by missionary physicians or to enumerate the scientific and other periodicals to which missionaries contributed. There was such a growing demand for scientific books that he could not spend a night in an interior city without being applied to by some of the best citizens to furnish them.

A large number of medical works have been written or translated by these missionaries. Dr. S. F. Green wrote thirty-two treatises in Tamil, including a volume on Obstetrics of 258 pages, a five-hundred-page manual of Surgery, still larger books on Anatomy, Physiology and Practice of Medicine, Eye Diseases, and several for popular use by mothers, etc.

Missionary doctors have sent home valuable specimens, illustrating medical botany, and †we believe that we are correct in stating that the supplies of snake poisons

---

* Missions and Science, p. 415.

† Up to date of publication the author has been unable to obtain absolute verification of this statement.

on which were based the experiments resulting in the manufacture of anti-venene were obtained through medical missionaries.

Cases which are rare and unusual in the home-country are often quite commonly met with in mission dispensaries and the missionary in love with his profession has an opportunity for enriching its knowledge, which is limited only by the leisure possible to give to such work. The missionary doctors are a power for civilization because of the information which they impart. The Chinese, for instance, are great quizzers, and the information imparted by conversation about means and methods used in Western lands must have an educational influence of no small importance.*

The service rendered to geography by missionaries has been a rich one, though in this case medical men, if Livingstone's splendid record be excepted, have had but a meagre share in what has been mainly achieved by the patient labor of other missionaries.   Mr. Colton, the famous mapmaker, says that there is hardly an exploration in any land which does not acknowledge its indebtedness to missionaries.   "Carl Ritter, the celebrated geographer, says he could not have written his great work but for the material furnished by missionaries."

The very difficulties under which work has to be performed by medical missionaries have often been fertile in inventiveness, as, for instance, the use of charred straw in Japan, and dressings of impregnated sawdust in Kashmir, as well as many clever instruments improvised from very simple materials.

The Example Has Stimulated Other Benevolent Undertakings. One of the most important humane efforts of the present century was directly due to the medical missionary work.   In its far-reaching results the Lady Dufferin Fund in India promises to be one of the great charities of that or any other land.   † "Its origin has all the elements of a touching romance.   In Punna, a city

* There are now medical journals published in India, China and Syria, and medical congresses have been held from time to time.

† Indika, p. 454.

about a hundred miles from Lucknow, there lives a native prince—the Maharajah. In 1881 his wife, the Maharani, was suffering from a serious and lingering disease. Her case was desperate. It is contrary to all tradition and propriety that a male physician should enter a zenana, or lady's chamber, and make such diagnosis as might secure intelligent treatment. Besides, no European physician, or indeed, any other Euporean, lived in Punna. The Prince had heard of Miss Beilby, a missionary physician, living in Lucknow, and he sent for her to attend his suffering wife. Miss Beilby not only responded to his imploring appeal, but remained with her patient for several weeks. The Rani was restored to health through the missionary's skill and care. Miss Beilby was soon to return to England . . . to take her degree in a medical college. On the morning of her departure from Punna, she called at the palace to say good-bye to her distinguished patient. The Rani was deeply affected. She had a great burden on her heart, and, dismissing all her ladies and attendants, said : ' You are going to England, and I want you to tell the Queen and Prince and Princess of Wales, and the men and women of England, what the women of India suffer when they are sick. Will you promise me?' The Rani was emphatic in confining her wishes to one thing : medical help for the suffering women of her dear India. But she was not willing that Miss Beilby should intrust the message to any one else ; she must deliver it herself to the good Queen of England. Miss Beilby explained the great difficulty of seeing the Queen in person and could give the Rani little encouragement that this could be brought to pass. When the Rani observed her readiness to do what she could, she asked Miss Beilby to write down the message at once. ' Write it small, Doctor Miss Sahib, for I want to put it into a locket and you are to wear this locket around your neck until you see our great Empress and give it to her yourself. You are not to send it through another.' "

The Queen granted an audience to Miss Beilby and took the little letter out of the locket and read it. She was deeply impressed. " We had no idea it was as bad as this. Something must be done for these poor creatures."

She sent a message of sympathy to the Rani and added:
" We should wish it generally known that we sympathize
with every effort made to relieve the suffering state of
the women of India." Lord Dufferin was then just about
to take up his duties of Governor-General for India. The
Queen saw Lady Dufferin and impressed on her the importance of making efforts to bring medical assistance to
India's suffering women.

So successful were her efforts that a year ago it was*
reported that there are eleven branches working under the
central committee, that 103 hospitals and dispensaries offi-
cered by women have been established, while in these hospitals, or in their own houses, 1,327,000 women received
medical aid from women during 1897. Twenty-eight
women, with British medical diplomas, seventy assistant
surgeons and seventy hospital assistants are employed in
the various zenana hospitals. The objects of the association are for the medical tuition and training of women as
doctors, hospital assistants, nurses and midwives, the
establishment of hospitals and dispensaries under the su-
perintendence of women. The association is purely philanthropic, though not missionary in any other sense. A
very large proportion, however, of the physicians, etc.,
have been drawn from Christian schools. The interest
excited in this noble and compassionate work has been
remarkable. Scholarships have been offered and funds
subscribed by many who would be untouched by a purely
religious undertaking.

Other benevolent acts have been stimulated from the
object lesson of Medical Missions. A few years ago a well-
to-do Parsee gentleman gave $50,000 to build a hospital for
women and children. † "An Indian woman placed at the
disposal of the government $60,000 for carrying on
women's medical work in the province of Bengal. Another has donated $6,000 for the erection of a hospital for
women."

One of the results of Dr. Howard's attendance on Li
Hung Chang's aged mother was a legacy left by her of
$1,000, which is stated to be the first bequest of a Chinese

---

* For these facts we are indebted to Dr. Jas. S. Dennis.

† Women in Missions, p. 169.

voman to Christian benevolence. Rev. Sidney Gulick, in
iis very thoughtful and suggestive book, " The Growth
)f the Kingdom of God," writes : " So sweet and reasona-
)le have these institutions and methods and principles
)een seen to be that all men praise and approve them.   So
important are many of them for the welfare of the com-
munity, that even governments do not 'esitate to contrib-
ite public money for their establishment and support.   Not
)nly the governments of Christian lands, but those of
ion-Christian lands, have quickly caught the spirit and
.re following the examples set them.

" Yet it still holds true that the great majority of those
vho give either their means, or especially themselves, to
)enevolent work among the poor and the wretched, the
'ile and the wicked, who established not only free hospi-
als for the sick, but rescue homes for the fallen, who la-
)or not only for temporal and physical comfort, but also
or the mental, moral and social improvement and welfare
)f the lower and vicious classes of society, are earnest
Christian men and women.   Yet the wide sympathy and
inancial help in its support that this form of the Chris-
ian's work and ideal find among non-Christians show
iow pervasive is the influence of Jesus, how far it has
pread beyond the limit of those who profess to be His
'isciples."

PREPARATION OF THE MEDICAL MISSIONARY

" It takes a soul
To move a body ; it takes a high-souled man
To move the masses even to a cleaner stye ;
It takes the ideal to blow an inch inside
The dust of the actual."

" I spoke as I saw,
I report as a man may of God's work—
All's love, yet all's law.
Now I lay down the judgeship He lent me,
Each faculty tasked ;
To perceive Him has gained an abyss
Where a dewdrop was asked."
—*Robt. Browning.*

' Life may be spent or invested : may be seed corn or devoured."

" He speaks not well who doth his time deplore,
Naming it new and little and obscure,
Ignoble and unfit for lofty deeds.
All times were modern in the times of them,
And this no more than others.
Do thy part
Here in the living day, as did the great
Who made the days immortal ! "
—*Richard Watson Gilder.*

V

PREPARATION OF THE MEDICAL MISSIONARY

The work of the lapidary is to enhance the reflecting power of the gem, and he is not content with polishing one side, but makes many facets so that from scores of angles the light breaks and burns. The Great Lapidary has made each precious stone in His treasury of amazing beauty from whichever side it is viewed. The piercing gleam from some facets near the setting is only seen on close inspection. The ministry of healing shines brightly upon us as we look at its spiritual service and tender winsomeness of compassion. The light is reflected from its very apex and almost every beam is caught and sent back to us with its clear and holy gleam. But by and by, as we look closer, we see that the lower angles have a glory all their own, though perhaps not quite so brilliant as the apex. The educational influence, the stimulation of benevolent enterprises and even sanitary reforms—these are the facets sometimes almost hidden, but which reflect the light all the same, when placed in the right point of view.

Every great life which has leaped out upon the world has taken generations to form. Every great national life has had back of it huge reservoirs of wise legislation and public spiritedness. It is no mean claim to make for Medical Missions that they have been instrumental in promoting a healthier—and therefore surely a holier—national life in the countries where they have been working.

It was said of Professor Owen that he could construct an entire skeleton from seeing a single bone of a prehistoric animal. We venture to think that the estimation in which a government holds the lives of its people, as evidenced by its care for the preservation of their health, prevention of disease and precautions against devastations by epidemics, might almost be taken as a rough gauge of the position they hold in the world of Christian Sociology, and from these facts might be built up a skeleton of its national well-being.

The field of influence is immense. The countries in which medical mis-

sionaries are working are, almost without exception, devoid of proper sanitation or the desire to enforce precautionary methods when threatened by wholesale death through epidemic illnesses.

A physician who has spent over twenty years in China says: "Their cities and towns are unspeakably filthy, many of their busy thoroughfares being but elongated cesspools. Every householder is at liberty to throw any kind of abominable refuse into the public street before his own door, and sanitary laws, if they exist, are neither understood nor enforced. The dwellings of the poor are minus everything that makes for comfort or conduces to health, and in times of sickness the condition of the sufferers, especially if they have the misfortune to be women, is extremely deplorable." " The nasal organs of the Chinese seem to be deficient in sensitiveness, and they endure with apparent impunity stenches that would make a European ill. Many of their rooms are dark and damp. The sewers in the cities are frequently foul, and often through superstitious notions are so constructed that the sewage collects in them instead of flowing off. Most of the villages in South China have pools into which all refuse matter is cast."

* " China is notorious for the entire neglect of proper sanitation. There is even a lively rivalry among its most important cities as to which deserves the prize for surpassing filthiness. Peking, the capital, seems to be by no means an unworthy candidate for the highest laurels in the contest, and has even been pronounced by competent judges as the dirtiest city on the face of the globe. 'Above all characteristics of Peking,' says Mr. Norman, ' one thing stands out in horrible prominence. Not to mention it would be wilfully to omit the most striking feature of the place. I mean its filth. It is the most horribly and

---

* Christian Missions and Social Progress. Dr. Jas. S. Dennis. Vol. I., p. 222.

indescribably filthy place that can be imagined; indeed, imagination must fall far short of the fact.' "

*Dr. Theodore Duka, an Indian army surgeon, says: " It is almost needless to enter upon a description of the sanitation of an Indian village, for there is a total absence of it. The huts composing the villages and hamlets are erected for the most part on flat land or on slightly elevated ground, exposed to the scorching sun and fiery winds, or drenched by rain. The people drink from the pond in which they bathe and in which their cattle wallow, surrounded by the refuse of their daily lives. The cattle consist of cows and buffaloes, occasionally of goats, donkeys and pigs. All live under the same roof and lie upon the ground beside their master and his family. There is hardly a window or an opening for ventilation."

Moslem lands are equally wanting in common sanitary knowledge. The annual pilgrimage to Mecca by thousands of Muhammedans is a menace to the whole world's health. It has been stated that every cholera visitation in any land during recent years has been plainly traceable to Mecca as its source. The crowding of the pilgrims, the water used for drinking, and every other condition seems to present an almost perfect combination for spreading contagion. The superstitious fears which are entertained in these lands of anything like scientific investigation for the purpose of public health is well illustrated by a quotation from †*The Lancet:* " The French Statistical Department, anxious to obtain definite information on certain matters from Turkish provinces, sent lists of questions to which they requested replies, to the various provincial Pashas. Certain of the questions were addressed to the Pasha of Damascus, and his replies ran as follows:

" Question: What is the death rate per thousand in your principal city?

" Answer: In Damascus it is the will of Allah that all must die; some died old, some young.

" Question: What is the annual number of births?

"Answer: We don't know; only God alone can say.

---

* Quoted from Christian Missions and Social Progress, Dr. Jas. S. Dennis. Vol. I., p. 219, 220.

† July 16, 1898.

"Question: Are the supplies of drinking water sufficient and of good quality?

"Answer: From the remotest period no one has ever died of thirst.

"Question: General remarks on the hygienic conditions of your city.

"Answer: Since Allah sent us Muhammed, His prophet, to purge the world with fire and sword, there has been a vast improvement. But there still remains much to do. Everywhere is opportunity to help and to reform. And now, my lamb of the West, cease your questioning, which can do no good either to you or to any one else. Man should not bother himself about matters which concern only God. Salem Aleikum!"

The medical missionary stands in a position of peculiar importance toward these things. He possesses the requisite professional knowledge, and, moreover, what is equally important, he has the confidence of the people. Who can help so well or with such authority as the physician who is already held in high esteem for his work's sake? The single act of vaccination has been the means of preserving thousands of lives. In Korea it is estimated by the native faculty that about 50 per cent. of the deaths are caused by smallpox. The doctors at a single mission hospital in China are stated to have vaccinated 25,000 patients in one year.*

In many parts of the East where a desert touches a piece of fertile ground, the sand is constantly drifting and making barren much soil which is capable of productiveness. Sometimes for a little while there is promise of fertility and then again comes the sand-drift, choking up life. But if there be some outjutting rock which will arrest the sand, then at last on the lee side of the rock there is a chance of some seed bringing forth a harvest of a hundred fold. The epidemics of disease in these lands are much like the sand blasts. They sweep across a land, stifling the life of helpless thousands and creating a sense of panic and fatalistic superstition. The missionary phy-

* The remarkable success of vaccination in these countries, where in the majority of cases the insanitary conditions remain as before, is surely a striking commentary on the statement made by the opponents of vaccination that the reduced mortality from smallpox is due to merely improved sanitation.

sician has been able again and again to arrest, in at least some measure, this drift and to stand " as an hiding place from the wind and a covert from the tempest, . . . as the shadow of a great rock in a weary land." He has been able to instil confidence in place of fear and to secure the adoption of suitable measures for meeting the epidemic and preventing its spread.

The comparative immunity of native Christians against such diseases as compared with other natives, was specially noted in connection with the plague in India in 1898. Careful, regular, cleanly and right living demonstrated its influence over health in a most noticeable manner.

The consideration of the high death rates in Oriental cities furnishes food for reflection. The annual mortality of infants and of women in labor is a call pathetic enough to stir our hearts as well as our brains. " Even in the City of Calcutta the infant death rate under one year of age in 1894 was 402 per 1000 and in 1893 it was 415." (Christian Missions and Social Progress. Dr. Jas. S. Dennis. Vol. I., page 220.) The death rate of infants under one year of age in the United States in census year ending May 31, 1890, was 225.9 per 1000 of total deaths, or almost half the proportion obtaining in Calcutta.

" The mortality of London has been reduced to about 20 per 1000 per annum. The mortality of most Oriental cities is over 45 per 1000, or more than double that of London." *

Considering the vastly reduced mortality to-day of surgical operations and the safe character of ordinary obstetric procedures it is probable that modern medical science under favorable conditions could remove or prevent more than half of the disease and pain suffered by peoples of mission lands. As they number more than half the population of the world, it will be seen what an immense burden of the world's physical woe might thus be lifted! Oh! for more men and women to stand and break the great drifts of sickness which blow from the deserts of disease; for men and women who will be a shadow of a great rock to their brothers and sisters in a weary land,

---

* Medical Missions at Home and Abroad. March, 1892. Page 86. See also *Student Volunteer*, Nov., 1895, p. 28, for interesting statistics.

who are scorched with the burning heat of fever and
tossed by the tempests of pain!

The law of the Kingdom is that to whom
Preparation of the much has been given, of him shall much
Profession. be required. *Noblesse oblige* is true of
princes in knowledge as well as princes in
rank. To-day the responsibility of the profession is
greater than on the day when organized foreign missionary
enterprise had its beginning. The past century has
wrought wonders in Medicine as well as in every other
branch of science.

In every age the instincts of brotherly love toward the
sick made demands which could not be denied by the followers of the God of Love. There was a challenge as
well as a gibe enshrined in Lucian's famous words concerning Christians. " Their Master," said he, " has per-
suaded them that they are all brothers." This fraternal
feeling was naturally manifested in an especial degree toward those who were sick and suffering, though the means
and requisite knowledge possessed at that early date were
but scanty for the alleviation of any but the simplest mal-
adies.

Christian physicians of this age have vastly greater
powers for demonstrating their brotherliness in this direc-
tion than had their predecessors. To the ignorant and
superstitious the achievements of hospital surgery seem
little short of miraculous. Without question they per-
form a somewhat similar function to that of the miracles
wrought by Christ in the early days of Christianity. They
call attention and by their very nature make the recipients
inclined to listen to the teaching with which they are accompanied.

" They soon learn that a religion of which such work
is the fruits cannot be altogether bad ; that a religion that
the foreign physician believes and that prompts him to
work among them under such disagreeable conditions,
and do for them things that their relatives are seldom willing to do, must have some reason in it. In short, they
hear the Gospel more regularly, and in a state of mind
produced by leisure, by freshness and by the spirit of the

place, better calculated to produce deep and lasting impressions than is usually the case at the church."

A hundred years ago Medical Missions to the heathen might have been organized. Great good would assuredly have resulted. But it would have been comparatively difficult in many lands to have demonstrated the superiority of Western Medicine over many of the methods in use among these peoples. Of course there would have been superiority observable and distinctly so ; but not of the spectacular nature which to-day is easy and which is such a power in breaking down prejudices and winning confidence. However superficially the history of Christianity be reviewed the impression is left vividly upon thought that for every great onward movement there has been a singular preparation of the world and of the agents through whom the world was to be impressed. The political conditions of the world's great powers at the advent of Christianity was a remarkable illustration of this. The preparation in this present century for world-wide missions is seen in the drawing together of all parts of the globe through rapid transit, railroad and steamship, telegraphy and postal systems, and the speedy propagation of thought by enormous hourly outputs from the printing press. Associate these material things with the revival of interest in foreign missions, exemplified by the concerts of prayer, foundation of missionary societies, rising interest among young people and the dedication of thousands of students and others to the cause of foreign missions, and it will be seen how the two forms of preparation meet at a focal point where they become capable of working in harmony for a great and widespread movement for the progress of the Kingdom of our Lord.

Just such a duplex preparation is seen in the world to-day for the wide establishment of Medical Missions in heathen lands.

Technical Preparation. A very brief survey will enable us to comprehend the wonderful technical armament which has become the property of the medical profession during this century of missions.

We have already alluded to one discovery which has so illumined the century—the discovery of the protection afforded against smallpox by vaccination. In our judgment, that one item of knowledge would be an almost priceless gift to bestow upon the rest of mankind. While it is to Jenner that we are indebted for this discovery it was many years before the scientific principles upon which its protection was based were clearly defined. Pasteur's splendid work on low forms of vegetable life not only put vaccination on a sure footing, but gave enormous impulse to an entirely new and very important department of science, which has shed light on scores of morbid processes, previously little understood. It was a stride of incalculable importance which was made when it was discovered that a large number of acute diseases were due to the presence in the body of some minute parasitic vegetation—germs or micro-organisms. This was but the beginning of still greater triumphs in the science of Bacteriology, or the study of these microscopic organisms.

The great complementary discovery to the above fact was made when it was found that many of these very virulent organisms manufactured a material which at last became inimical to their own existence. Not only has it thus been possible to identify the actual morbific agent of a disease, but also to single out and apply the remedial product in the form of " anti-toxins."*

To give but one example (and that perhaps the most striking) of the reduction of deaths through this new method of treatment, we would instance the use of the diphtheria anti-toxin. This has only been before the profession as a whole since the fall of 1894. The reduction of mortality through its use has been one of the modern triumphs of therapeutics. In some hospitals the number of deaths occurring has been considerably less than one-third the mortality previous to its use. That is to say, that out of every 100 persons who formerly would have died, sixty-six lives are now saved.† Research along similar lines has yielded results of varying degrees of value in the treatment of cholera, bubonic plague, hydrophobia,

---

* This is an exceedingly rough and popular statement of the facts, and is not scientifically precisely the case in many instances.

† Medical readers may be referred to very interesting and instructive articles in Annual of Gynaec. and Pediat., No. 7, 1897, by F. L. Morse, and *Brit. Med. Journal*, Jan. 28, 1899, p. 197.

and tuberculosis. It is even claimed already that it has yielded light on the origin of cancer, though this latter claim has by no means been established as a scientific fact.*

But perhaps the greatest contribution that Bacteriology has made to the realm of practical Medicine has been its surgical aspect. The work of Pasteur, Tyndall and Lister is now almost classical and finds its popular expression in the term " listerism." These scientists each contributed to the others' work, which led Lister at last to the discovery that the inflammation of surgical wounds was due to the fermentative processes of these minute organisms. That discovery made, it was but a step to the finding that certain chemical solutions were poisonous to these germ-bodies. Lister found that by using solutions of certain germicidal chemicals the putrefactive changes could be controlled or abolished. Such a discovery has done nothing less than revolutionize the whole of surgical procedure. Lord Lister, it has been stated, has probably, by means of this discovery, saved more lives and mitigated more suffering than any man living in this or any past generation. This seems excessive tribute, and yet when one compares the frightful death rate in the past in serious operations with that of the present day, one realizes it is probably the statement of an actual fact.† The enunciation of antiseptic and aseptic principles has not only widened our scope, but has permitted the entrance into surgical fields unthought of in our fathers' time.

The safety and brilliancy of cranial and abdominal operations lies as a heavy hand of responsibility upon us to devote our securer knowledge and safer manipulative skill to this supremest and noblest service of God among those to whom we can be an agent of physical salvation and a messenger of spiritual hope. Many injuries no longer form a *noli me tangere* to the surgeon which before were cause of intense anxiety as to whether he was justified in attempting surgical alleviation. But even this priceless boon could not have been fully appropriated, if

---

* See *Practitioner*, April, 1899, for latest views of American and British authorities

† " Eighty per cent. of all wounds treated " in Nussbaum's clinic in Munich " were attacked by hospital gangrene. Erysipelas was the order of the day to such an extent that its occurrence could almost have been looked upon as the normal course." (Deutsche Zeitschrift für Chirurgie. 1877.)

there had not also come to mankind the discovery of anæsthetics in this century. We hardly know which is the greater gift; their benefits seem to interact one upon the other, and each of these twin discoveries is indispensable to modern surgery. Yet perhaps the palm is to be accorded to the sister of sleep. It is now easy for the surgeon to conduct his investigation into regions which would have been impossible but for the benign influence of the " deep and painless slumber " induced by chloroform or ether. And we would give the palm the more readily to the discovery of anæsthetics when we gratefully remember its special service to motherhood in the " hour of trial."

The use of chloroform is always a wonder in a Medical Mission hospital. The performance of painful procedures without the patient feeling anything, is a new token to a Chinaman of the wonderful power of the foreign doctor.

This century has been rich in its inventiveness, which has made the discovery and investigation of disease far more definite and exact. The stethoscope has been a sixth sense to the physician in his knowledge of chest and heart diseases, and even now its capabilities are annually being enlarged and improved upon. The ophthalmoscope is to the surgeon what the photographic plate is to the astronomer—a piercing eye which can see further and find more than could unaided vision. The laryngoscope and clinical thermometer are other outstanding products of scientific Medicine.

The discovery of oxygen at the close of the eighteenth century and the demonstration of its relation to the blood, the manufacture of quinine, strychnine, iodides, bromides, and a score of other " ines " and " ides " have all been of the past one hundred years.

The work of Buffon, Cuvier, Hunter, Owen and Darwin in natural history has laid a sure foundation for biological data and the principles deducible from them. The first sanitary commissions were instituted in 1838 and 1844, and from those commissions went out impulses for betterment of the public health of the people which have been felt in nearly every civilized land.

" Nursing, from time immemorial, the tending of

the sick as a work of pure charity, has been carried on by religious communities. It is within our own times that the science and art of nursing have risen to their high standard, combining the highest motives with the highest efficiency, thanks to the completeness and the discipline of hospital training and to the advanced teaching of the physician and surgeon. To Miss Florence Nightingale's noble service is this specially due."

The treatment of the insane has been humanized since Pinel began his investigations in France. It was strange how long even in Christian lands the superstitions remained as to those mentally afflicted being possessed by evil spirits, or at least being " uncanny " and to be dreaded and treated with cruelty. Even physicians publicly advocated such treatment. Happily a party possessing such opinions no longer exists among the members of the profession to-day, and we can ask with Hans Breitmann, " Vhere ish dot barty now? " without fear of its discovery in any corner of our land.

We have enumerated but a very few of the advances of Medicine in this century. It would have been a pleasant task to review it with some fullness, believing as we do that we are but recording events which conspire together in making this era the most favorable ever known for the prosecution of Medical Missions. This, then, is our heritage to-day! What are we doing with it? We are to-day as men holding ten talents of latent power, and God does not expect from us the smaller services of two-talent men. Whether we stay at home or abroad, we are weighted with responsibility to invest all for the glory of God, Who bestowed them.

Never before in the history of Medicine has the Christian physician had at his command such immense resources. Are the benefits of these resources to be confined to about one hundred million people of America and Europe? Are the sufferings of two-thirds of the world's population to go untended? Is maternity to be a dreaded nightmare to our sisters in India and China, Persia and Africa, when the women of our own lands are tended with care and considerateness? Are thousands to lose their sight each year because there are no surgeons at hand to couch cataracts?

The answer to all this is far deeper than the mere claims made upon us because of the wonderful preparedness of the profession. Once more we may say that the answer spells itself out in love to God. When the fire from off the altar of love touches our lips, shall we not be constrained to cry, " Here am I ; send me " ?

Spiritual Preparation of the Profession. The preparation of the profession is not technical alone; it is spiritual. For many generations there·have been men who illumined the profession not by their medical work alone, but because they stood enrolled as humble followers of Jesus Christ. The names of Haller and Boerhaave, Cheselden and Paré, Sydenham and Abercrombie, and in later days, Simpson, the discoverer of chloroform; Sir Andrew Clark, " the prince of physicians and one of the noblest of men," and a host of others, will be remembered for their deep personal faith as well as their scientific attainments.* To-day, however, this spiritual phalanx is vaster and stands more compact in the army of medical practitioners than ever before.

A man of great experience and keen insight told the author that it was hard, forty years ago, to find Christian doctors in England ; now they are numerous. The spiritual awakening among medical students is even more remarkable. Thousands are to-day enrolled in Christian associations in medical colleges in North America and Europe. This has practically been entirely the growth of the past fifteen years. The medical students who have decided to become foreign missionaries during the past eight years may be counted by hundreds.

What does this preparation, both technical and spiritual, mean ? Does it not mean that the Spirit of God would lead forth a band of men and women who have studied in the schools of Western Medicine, into a fuller, larger, holier and nobler service, in lands whose need sorely cries out for helpers and healers, and whose spiritual darkness requires the rising of the Sun of Righteousness if the black clouds of ignorance, superstition, cruelty and sin are to be rolled back and a fairer day is to dawn?

---

* We have purposely omitted names of any living physicians. It would be easy to compile a very long list of such.

AN APPEAL

" I cared not where or how I lived, or what hardships I went through, so that I could but gain souls to Christ. While I was asleep I dreamed of these things, and when I waked the first thing I thought of was this great work. I longed to be a flame of fire, continually glowing in the service of God and building up Christ's Kingdom to my latest, my dying moments."

—David Brainerd.

" To the spirit select there is no choice.
He cannot say, This will I do or that.

. . . .
A hand is stretched to him from out the dark,
Which grasping without question, he is led
Where there is work that he must do for God.

. . . .
To the tough hearts that pioneer their kind
And break a pathway to those unknown realms
That in the earth's broad shadow lie enthralled,
Endurance is the crowning quality,
And patience all the passion of great hearts."

—James Russell Lowell.

" The day is short, and the task is great, and the workmen are sluggish, and the reward is much, and the Master of the House is urgent."

—Rabbi Tarphon.

" Wanted—men :
Not systems fit and wise,
Not faiths with rigid eyes,
Not wealth in mountain piles,
Not power with gracious smiles,
Not even the potent pen :
Wanted—MEN."

VI

AN APPEAL

The work of the medical missionary is many-sided. It is not bisected into two parts designated as spiritual and medical. Like the shield, it has two sides, but it is a whole—a spiritual whole. The medical missionary goes as a spiritual agent to do spiritual work and that motive dominates his task just as truly when he is amputating a limb as when he is lending a hand to some poor fellow battling and beaten with the waves of sin. Like the water filling the empty vase the work takes on different forms according to the delimiting surroundings.

The Day's Work.

It might roughly be enumerated as follows : (1) Work among patients in hospital, hospital employees and among students or nurses. This would include a simple service every morning in the wards, the loaning of books and tracts and as much personal conversation with patients as possible. This is needed to deepen the feeling in patients that the doctor cares for their higher natures far more deeply than for their mere physical needs ; that they are not " cases," but brothers and sisters of himself. It is needed also to find out how far his more public exhortations are being understood and to very simply explain the real meaning of these strange doctrines which are so new and often so incomprehensible to their minds. Sometimes a special meeting is held each week for detailed explanation of the Bible and often a prayer meeting for the Christians is a regular feature of a mission hospital. This is probably the aspect of work which bears the greatest fruitage ; it is more costly in time and sympathy and therefore is more productive. In a very real spiritual sense it is axiomatic that " whatsoever a man soweth, that shall he also reap."

(2) Service for the out-patients on receiving days. As a rule the out-patients are gathered together into two halls or rooms, one for men and one for women.   A Christian service of a very simple nature is held previous to each company being seen by the physician. This service is usually conducted by the doctor, and is followed up by native evangelists and Bible-women. In some missions each patient is given a ticket with a number upon it and a text of Scripture.   The number allows them to proceed in the order in which they arrived. This impartiality is in itself a striking lesson, as difference of rank is thus neglected, and the rich or high caste are not permitted to take precedence over the poor or pariah.

(3) House-to-house visitation is partly engaged in at the call of those natives in need of medical aid.   It is also done among those who have left the hospital after treatment.   Some very valuable results have accrued from this outside visiting.   Often it has been to some high official's house, and has afforded a splendid opportunity for introducing the Gospel to those who would be reached in no other way.   The majority of medical missionaries, however, seem inclined to believe that this outside work should not be cultivated, as taking away time from the sphere of work in the hospital which is usually deemed most fruitful.   Occasionally, however, it is found eminently expedient to embrace such opportunities.   An important addition to outside calls is that often made by the presence of other missionary families needing attendance, either in or near the Medical Mission.

(4) Medical itinerating.   The value of this form of effort varies greatly according to the country.   Dr. Grace N. Kimball, of Van, Turkey, so well known for her brave services at the time of the Armenian massacres, speaks of this form of effort as being almost unworthy of the time expended : "A medical missionary goes on an itinerating trip, visiting a large number of villages, staying a day or two in each, seeing all the multitude who come, free, giving each a dose of medicine, preaching the Gospel and passing on.   This makes a very telling letter to the missionary magazine, yields a great and fascinating excitement to the missionary . . . and yet the price paid for this has

been a lavish expenditure of physical strength on the
part of the medical missionary and of medicines and other
medical adjutants, much of which can legitimately be
considered thrown away."

On the other hand, there is a chorus of praise accorded by missionaries in other parts of the world to this
plan, which on the surface harmonizes so nearly with
that adopted by Christ. Sometimes the spectacular demonstration of minor surgical procedures is enough to
stimulate further inquiry into the doctrines preached and
to bring other and more serious medical cases from distant villages to the hospital. These returning to their
own homes, become propagating centres of Christianity.
It also makes a profound difference whether there are native workers in the districts visited to follow up the work.
In Japan, such medical touring has had to be done in co-
operation with the local physicians and copies of the pre-
scriptions given handed to him, on account of the legal requirements regulating medical practice in that Empire.
Itinerating is often of value as a help to little churches
distant and scattered, and cheers on the natives who may be
working among their countrymen. It is the means also
of leaving the permanent influence of books and leaflets
in the hands of very many who have listened to the
preaching of the missionary physician.

(5) In addition to all the above, comes the actual medical work of the physician. It consists in seeing patients,
prescribing, operating, dressing their wounds and very
often dispensing medicines, making and adapting apparatus, as well as the exacting work of recording cases, or-
dering drugs and keeping accounts. A medical missionary may also have on his hands the training of several
young men as dressers or as qualified practitioners. No
wonder that a man needs to be well qualified where he has
to be his own anæsthetist, dresser, clerk, hospital archi-
tect, and superintendent, dispenser and compounder, nurse
and house surgeon!

Diseases Many of the diseases dealt with find their coun-
Prevalent. terpart in any large hospital at home, yet there
are others which are frequent in these lands
and are excessively rare among ourselves.

A graphic and very representative picture of a physician's daily ward visit is given by Dr. James A. Greig, of
Kirin, Manchuria: " In the early hours of the morning
we pay our visit to the wards to see how our patients are
getting on. We can accommodate between forty and
fifty, and usually the wards are nearly full. As I enter
a ward the word goes round, ' Ta-fu lai la! Ta-fu lai la!'
' The Doctor has come! The doctor has come!' and
many pale faces turn toward me, and anxious hearts eagerly await my words of advice, of cheer or of warning.
As each temperature chart is examined and surgical dressing changed, one realizes the enormous power we in Western lands have received for doing good and relieving suffering in the dark places of the earth. How delightful to
watch the return of health to the frame wasted by disease,
and to see the cruel, fiery hand of ophthalmia arrested ere
the sunshine of life dies out and the darkness of incurable
blindness sets in. To soothe the fevered brow and relieve the racking pain is at once our privilege and reward.
That bronzed and emaciated fellow is a martyr to tubercu-
lar disease. One of his limbs had to be removed and several other operations had subsequently to be performed.
He has had a long and trying time of it, but now he is beginning to mend. Months ago he would have died in a
miserable dirty hovel but for the kindly help he has received.
    " The man in the second bed from the door was
brought to us from a town a hundred miles away, suffering from a form of cancer. The growth has been com-
pletely excised, and the wound has now healed. He has
had a severe struggle breaking off the opium habit, which
he had acquired while seeking relief from pain. He has
succeeded in stopping the use of the drug, and is returning home in a day or two. The lad in yonder cot broke
his thigh when playing with some comrades. As he calm-
ly slept under an anæsthetic, we set and comfortably band-
aged his limb in a rigid apparatus, and now it is only a
matter of time, and without deformity or lameness he will
be able to romp and play once more.
    " These three young men, with their arms in slings,
were injured in the arsenal. The making of silver coins,

which has recently been instituted, has caused a number of accidents, as the machinery is new and not well understood. These men were injured in this department.

" That little boy was dreadfully burnt about the neck and chest while making percussion caps. For some nights we feared he would not survive, but he did. Then his eyes were our chief anxiety. He begged and prayed us to give him back his sight. After many weeks one of his eyes was restored, and he is very happy over it.

" The sallow, careworn-looking man next the window is, I fear, beyond hope of cure. He came to us with very advanced bone disease, and although he has had two operations under chloroform, and everything has been done that our skill could suggest, his chance is not good. He is an only son, and his old father bends over him day by day with all his paternal tenderness, but there is little improvement. But most of our cases do well, and it is glad work."

Skin diseases are frequent and doubtless the uncleanly habits of the people have a large place as the *causa causans* of many of them. Eye troubles of all kinds abound. A fruitful source of disease of the eyelids in China is the custom of barbers turning them over and " cleaning " them. After this process the eye is found to be inflamed, which being considered proof of insufficient cleaning of the lids, the practice is persisted in, leading to serious and often permanent injury.

The poor food, the use of salt provisions and the general irregularity in eating cause a great deal of dyspepsia in certain countries. Inflammatory diseases are not so common with the Chinese as in our own lands, and their lymphatic constitutions make them unexcelled as patients in bearing pain of operations. Leprosy is prevalent in India and China ; malarial fevers, tumors, and epidemic illnesses are common in the majority of Medical Mission lands.

Difficulties. Some of the difficulties encountered in the work are due to ignorance or superstition which in time will disappear.

Impatience is not peculiar to these lands ; every hospi-

tal surgeon at home has had sad experience in dealing
with it. But united with ignorance it is perhaps more un-
manageable. As an example, we might instance a case
that Dr. Kenneth Mackenzie received into his hospital—a
man with fracture of the thigh-bone. " It had been re-
peatedly explained to him that he must on no account remove the splint and appliances and that time would be required to effect a complete cure ; but at the end of a week,
seeing no manifest improvement, his friends removed the
bandages and splint and carried him off."

The *meddlesomeness* of patients and their desire to ex-
hibit their wounds to friends and relatives cause many
a heart burning to the surgeon who has just dressed the
wound with every precaution of " surgical cleanliness."
Again and again has a patient lost an eye through subsequent inflammation from caring nothing for the warning
not to touch the dressing, repeated over and over by the
physician.

Injurious dietary is another difficulty even with hospital patients. In mission hospitals in China one or more
friends of the patient come to nurse him. It requires excessive vigilance on the part of the doctor to prevent injurious food being administered surreptitiously by friends.
A typhoid case on the high road to recovery has been
hurried to a fatal termination through such mistaken kindness of so-called friends.

These are but samples of the thousand and one petty
troubles of a missionary doctor. " What with the strain
of grasping the essential details of every case, and choos-
ing the appropriate remedy for each, the cramped posture
while bending over and operating on some surgical case,
and the necessity during all of seeing everything that is
going on and maintaining order, it is no wonder if one is
tempted to lose patience. What superhuman patience
must Christ have had! Thronged by multitudes who
came only to witness miracles, worried about a thousand
trifling ailments, and where not trifling or fanciful, about
sickness, to a great extent the direct consequences of lust,
dirt and greed, argued with by sneering priests and understood by none. We speak of following Him ; we speak

of Christlike work; but, oh! how different is the spirit and power of its performance."*

Still deeper difficulties are the malicious reports which may be placarded about and which have to be lived down; and the indifference of patients to the spiritual side of the work—coming for what they can get of physical benefit, but caring nothing for the call of the Great Shepherd of Souls to return home to the Father's house.

> " Into a desolate land
> White with the driven snow,
> Into a weary land
> (Their) truant footsteps go.
> Yet doth Thy care, O Father,
> Even Thy wanderers keep ;
> Still doth Thy love, O Shepherd,
> Follow Thy sheep."

How the chilling apathy of patients must oppress the physician! The enormous inertia to be overcome, even by such favorable means as Medicine, must sometimes almost crowd optimism out of the field ; and hope, and even faith, are beleaguered on every side by the crushing weight of difficulty. But the sun shines again and gratitude and humble following of Jesus Christ is the glorious result in the lives of many others; and that is reward enough.

The author is quite unable to pronounce on **Qualifications Needed.** the qualifications necessary for such work as the foregoing pages indicate. The remarks following are almost wholly drawn from those who are able to speak with authority.†

1. There can be no question that the foremost qualification needed for a medical missionary is that *he should be a sincere and earnest follower of Jesus Christ.* It would seem superfluous to write this down. Yet from the author's personal knowledge it is a most needed statement. Not once or twice, but many times, have medical students spoken to us about becoming medical missionaries when

---

* Dr. Arthur Neve in *Medical Missions at Home and Abroad.* March, 1889 Page 265.

† This section is largely adapted from Chap. 10 of " The Medical Mission." Dr. W. J. Wanless. 1898.

they freely acknowledged that they were not followers of
Jesus Christ.   We would bid God-speed to every man or
woman who will help to heal the world's heart disease
from whatever motive.   We rejoice in every humanitarian and humane effort for the alleviation of suffering,
and we wish that such efforts might be extended and aug-
mented in these needy lands ; but we would nevertheless
remind ourselves of the difference between such works of
philanthropy and the work of healing the sick in the name
and for the sake of the Lord Jesus and with the clearly defined purpose of letting the work of healing be subordinate
and introductory to preaching the Good Tidings of the
love of God and salvation from sin.

As a visitor stands in the busiest part of the City of
London at noonday he hears the peal of a score of church
bells ringing out the hour.   Louder than all the chimes of
London booms out the great bell of St. Paul's Cathedral,
on whose rim, suspended high above all other bells, are
engraved the words, " Woe is unto me if I preach not the
Gospel."   A hundred lesser bells are ringing out the messages of altruism, humanity and the brotherhood of man,
but far higher than these peals out the glorious Gospel of
our Lord Jesus Christ, a Gospel setting forth not an ideal
alone, but bringing a strength into the individual life for
the attainment of that ideal.

It is this ideal for which the medical missionary lives.
If men and women are going with this message, it is
requisite that they know very personally the Saviour of
whom they speak and experience in daily life the salvation
which they, as ambassadors, offer to others.   It is true
that much of the work is what is termed secular and rou-
tine.   That is greater reason for the medical missionary
being thoroughly furnished unto every good work, and
having all the checks and stimuli to be found from a life
hid with Christ in God.

2. *He should be a good doctor.*—" In the mission field
he will be thrown back on his own resources.   He is often
alone in face of the gravest responsibilities.   He is not
sustained by an educated public sentiment which will insure for him an enlightened and charitable view of all that
he does.   He is surrounded by envious **charlatans, who**

will spare no efforts to injure him by detraction and mis-
representation. In such circumstances he has need of all
the knowledge and skill furnished by a thorough medical
training, of all the resources of a well-balanced mind and
a courageous heart. His failure will not injure him alone.
His success will advance the cause of Christ." *

Professional efficiency does not necessarily mean professional celebrity. It means a thorough, all-round medical education, such as any diligent student may secure by
a four to five years' curriculum in a high-grade medical
college. A year's hospital or post-graduate experience will
be a very valuable addition to such a course. In any case sufficient knowledge should be gained to insure personal confidence and progressive efficiency when on the field. The large
amount of surgical and ophthalmic work to be done will
naturally suggest those subjects as worthy of specialization
in the year after graduation. Do not let any think that their
brilliant talents will be wasted and find no adequate field
of effort in this work. The highest and best is too low
and too poor for the Master's royal service.

Harold Schofield did not throw away his talents, which
had won him $7,000 in prizes and scholarships, when he
went out to China and lived and died there inside of a
decade. China is still feeling the vibration of that heart
beat; the stray snatches of music in scores of lives have
reset themselves into a scheme of a higher and more con-
sistent harmony, through the controlling influence of his
life's song.

Is it a light or irresponsible work that any should
fancy the best is far too good for use where the remuneration is but that of a satisfied conscience and a heart filled
with the quiet joy of being serviceable? Ruskin says
finely, " It is an incomparably less guilty form of robbing,
to cut a purse out of a man's pocket than to take it out of
his hand on the understanding that you are to steer his
ship up channel, when you do not know the soundings.
The medical man has precious human ships to steer up the
channel of disease, which is studded with rocks and shoals,
to the harbor of health, and heavy and stringent is the obligation that rests upon him to make himself intimately ac-

* G. E. Post, M.D., Beyrout,

quainted with its pathological soundings; only by assiduous and prolonged study can he hope faithfully to prepare himself for his work."

3. *Good health.*—Clearly the work is intense with heavy responsibilities. Physically and mentally he is ever subject to an exceptional strain. "Add to this the enervation of a foreign climate and the occasion for sound health is at once manifest. The student who is able at the present time to endure the pressure of a three or four years' medical course in addition to a preliminary education without impairment of his general health or nervous system, will promise well for successful endurance on the foreign field. It is not always necessary that a student possess an athletic physique or robust appearance, but the work does call for the power of endurance, a temperament neither nervous nor phlegmatic, a disposition devoid of irritability, but hopeful and courageous. An extraordinarily healthy appearance, though desirable, is not always demanded, but good staying qualities are indispensable. It is not always those who apparently are best fitted to withstand the strain of work and climate that actually enjoy the best health. *Indeed the reverse is often the case. A previous record of good health under continued mental pressure and physical trial at home augurs well for continued good health abroad, and is probably the best guide in the decision as regards bodily endurance abroad.**

4. It is desirable, though not essential, that the missionary doctor be *apt to teach.* " He is often the entering wedge for others, he is a buttress to his evangelistic colleagues, he is often preaching best when practising in the name and spirit of Christ. But if he has also the gift of speech, not necessarily of making speeches, but of apt, ready use of his opportunities by well-chosen words of sympathy, advice, rebuke, instruction and inspiration, his influence will be two-fold. For this purpose he should be specially grounded in the Scriptures and imbued with the spirit of prayer. As his acumen in diagnosis is only a prelude to his skill in prescribing the medicine or performing the operation which offers hope and life, so

---

* The Medical Mission. W. J. Wanless. Pages 72, 73. The italics are our own.

should his spiritual insight into the wants of his patient be a preparation for the words which may reform his life and save his soul."

Appeal. We have seen the need of the heathen world; we have realized a little of the value of Medical Missions, directly, indirectly and reflexly. What are we going to do? Shall we stay here in America, where there is a physician to about every 550 people, or shall we go to India, where it is estimated by no less an authority than Sir William Moore that not 5 per cent. of the population is at present reached by medical aid? It is stated that even in Calcutta, one of the best medically equipped cities of Asia, three-fifths of the people have no medical attendance in their last illness. And this in India, with her government hospitals and dispensaries and her magnificent Lady Dufferin Scheme of relief. Do we not hear the mute appeal from China? In North America there are considerably more than 4,000 physicians to every two and a half million people. China has but one medical missionary for a similar population, though her need is a hundred-fold greater.*

We have in addition to the physicians our great hospitals, nursing institutions, orphanages, convalescent homes, and homes for the incurable and dying. We have the knowledge of the laws of health, hygiene and sanitation. If recovery of a friend is unsatisfactory, there are specialists and consultants by the score in our great cities, whose help may be secured. Skilled nurses are obtain-

---

* "The following statistics include data which have been verified and may stand as a fairly approximate—not absolutely complete—representation of the philanthropic agencies of missions. The total of medical missionaries at present is 680; of this number 470 are men and 210 women. There are 45 medical schools and classes, with 382 male and 79 female students—making a total of 461. There are 21 training schools for nurses, with 146 pupils. Neither of these statements includes 240 female medical students now in training as physicians, nurses and hospital assistants, under the care of the Lady Dufferin Association in India. There are 348 hospitals and 774 dispensaries. Exact statements as to the number of patients annually treated have been obtained from 293 hospitals and 661 dispensaries, the total patients recorded in these returns being 2,009,970, representing 5,087,169 treatments. If we make a proportionate estimate for the 55 hospitals and 113 dispensaries from which reports of the number of patients have not as yet been received, the sum total of those annually treated will be not far from 2,500,000. If we allow an average of three separate visits or treatments for each patient the total of annual treatments will be 7,500,000. There are 97 leper asylums, homes and settlements, with 5453 inmates, of whom 1987 are Christians. There are 227 orphan and foundling asylums, with 14,695 inmates." (Christian Missions and Social Progress, Vol. II. Dr. Jas. S. Dennis.)

able at an hour's notice, and the presence of sickness in
our midst draws forth at once the tenderest of care and
sweetest forethought from relatives and friends. It does
not state the case therefore to look merely at the lack
of doctors alone, though that is to pronounce China's need
as four thousand times greater than our own. Her cry
is loud and long and so few hear or heed.

Accountability is equal to capability. Our training in
the school of sympathy, our knowledge of the remedial
agents of disease and our personal realization of the need
of sin for a supernatural salvation constitute a call from
God. Coal on a great vessel is only so much ballast until turned into steam. So these talents given by the Spirit
of God are only ballast in our lives till employed for the
highest purposes for which they were granted.

If the reader is a follower of Christ, it is to Christ that
he must look for instruction as to his life-work. We have
no right to drift into it through forces of environment or
heredity; nor have we a right to choose it because it
pleases our scientific tastes or because it offers a congenial
employment with pecuniary remuneration, and social
status. Before all or any of these things must be heard
the definite asking of God for the light of His plan for our
lives. " Every man's life is a plan of God," and until that
is seen let us not step into our life-work. Emerson says
that the great crises of life are not marriages and deaths,
but some afternoon at the turn of a road when your life
finds new thoughts and impulses. Such crises occur as
a man hears the strong crying of a great need unrealized
before, and which he is conscious could be met by his own
life service.

In some great hospitals a bell is rung each time an accident case arrives. Can you not fancy—and after all it
is not very largely imagination—that you hear the sound
of that accident bell, reverberating round the world?

Did you hear it just now—it was from China that the
sound came. A poor Chinaman has fallen from a tree
and injured himself. A crowd gathers round; they gaze
and laugh at his sufferings, and when they have had
enough, move off and leave him to die.* Exaggeration,

---

* This, and each of the following cases, is a *fact*.

·you say? No, sober truth; there is no Red Cross man there to take him to a hospital, no ambulance to carry him, no hospital to which to take him. If he cannot move, his fellow countrymen will not help him. He will lie there and die.

The bell is ringing in India. A boy has broken his leg. A string will be tied tightly round the fractured limb until at last gangrene sets in and a foreign doctor is sent for to amputate in order to save his life.

The sound of the bell in Persia is wafted to us across the great plains and mountains of Asia. It tells of a woman in the hour of nature's sorest trial. The husband is by and also a medical missionary. " No, thanks; you needn't trouble to operate; it's only a wife; I can easily get a new one, and I want a change."

Now, it is booming and tolling in Africa, for a child in convulsions. What is to be done? A red-hot iron is pressed to the skull till a hole is burned down to the brain to let the demons out. Why not, it's only a *girl;* let her die.

The bell sounds clearer and nearer now; it is ringing in a city of America. Some poor fellow has had his arm wrenched off by machinery. What is going to be done? He is taken to a hospital, an interne or house surgeon sees him, a nurse is there to carefully tend him, to-morrow he will be seen by a visiting surgeon. If it is an operation, it will be done under an anæsthetic.

It rings again in the home land; this time a child is sick. If it is a poor child, our splendid children's hospitals are open for its reception. If it is the child of rich parents, the nursery will be made bright, relatives and friends will bring flowers and toys and fruit; a trained nurse will be y to relieve every discomfort and a physi-· cian stands there doing his noble best for the little life which hovers on the borderland of life and death. And all for a little child.

It rings once more a loud and urgent summons. A sister in the pangs of motherhood. Thank God, there are gentle voices, hushed footsteps, the skill and care of doctor and nurse—all these are immediately and as a simple

right bestowed on her and on the little life for whose sake
she is in sore travail. Thank God it is so!

Brothers, and sisters, why this difference? Has the
voice of Jesus become so feeble that we cannot hear it?
Or, are we standing out of hearing distance? These are
no imaginary instances; they are real. Thousands are
dying every day because Christian physicians have pre-
ferred to stay at home and fight for a living with fellow
practitioners, instead of forsaking all to follow our Lord
and fight the battles of the King. Do you think that if
you go there will be a single case untended, a single accident untreated? You know that scores are pressing and
pushing behind you and will take up all the work that you
lay down. But over there—if you neglect the opportunity of this love-service, they must suffer in unrelieved
pain, and if death occur, there will be no comforter at
hand to point them to the Guide of the shadowed valley.
Not because of the needs of the heathen, not because of
their ignorance or superstition or cruelty, but for the sake
of Him Who loved us and gave Himself for us, shall we
not go?

Duty, opportunity, altruism are in themselves motives
insufficient to impel us forward with fire and fervor which
shall stand the strain and stress of disappointment and in-
gratitude and fatigue. There is but one motive powerful
enough; it is the greatest thing in the world—LOVE.

What holds us back? A silver dollar, a medical di-
ploma, a life of comfort or distinction—these may loom so
large in our vision as to shut out the face of Jesus as He
bends in compassion over the suffering ones and turns to
us with that piercing look and says, " Inasmuch—inasmuch—as ye did it not . . . ye did it not unto Me."
If He, the Master of men, were here on earth to-day and
wandered into one of our out-patient departments, would
not we esteem it a royal privilege to bind up a finger of the
Lord Christ, to be even for once His court physician?

And this is the privilege to which He invites us, if we
would hear some day those other words: " Inasmuch as
ye did it unto one of these, My brethren, even these least,
ye did it unto Me."

"God said : 'Break thou these yokes ! Undo
These heavy burdens ! I ordain
A work to last thy whole life through—
A ministry of strife and pain.

"'Forego thy dreams of lettered ease ;
Put thou the scholar's promise by ;
The rights of man are more than these.'
He heard and answered, 'Here am I.' "*

* The author is indebted for some of the illustrations used in this last section to " A
Cry of Pain," by Miss Garvock, Church Missionary Society, England.

NOTE.—The literature on Medical Missions is not large. Much of it is in the form of biographies of missionary physicians. It does not, therefore, provide a great deal of available material for the study of the subject *per se.*

With the exception of biographies, the literature is also for the most part contained in magazines and periodicals. It would obviously be useless to give numerous references to denominational magazines, as very few colleges have the past files of many missionary periodicals issued by the numerous boards.

For these reasons it is suggested that each study class secure and use three pamphlets along with the foregoing chapters.

These pamphlets are :

The Medical Mission, by W. J. Wanless, M.D.

The Medical Arm of the Missionary Service. (A. B. C.)

Murdered Millions, by Geo, D. Dowkontt, M.D.

Files should, if possible, be obtained of the following medical missionary magazines :

The Double Cross and Medical Missionary Record.

Medical Missions at Home and Abroad.

Frequent reference will also be made to "Medical Missions : Their Place and Power," by J. Lowe.

ADDITIONAL READINGS FOR CHAPTER I.

BARNES, I. II. : Behind the Great Wall. 1896. pp. 113, 114.

BIRD-BISHOP, ISABELLA : Korea and Her Neighbours. 1897. pp. 202-204.

Double Cross, The : Oct., 1896, p. 216 ; March, 1897, p. 59 ; April, 1898, pp. 115, 119.

DENNIS, JAMES S. : Christian Missions and Social Progress. 1898. pp. 187-189, 191, 193, 198.

DOUGLAS, R. K. : Society in China. 1894. p. 115.

DOWKONTT, GEO. D. : Murdered Millions. 1897 ed. pp. 20-25, 27, 59-61.

GALE, J. S. : Korean Sketches. 1898. pp. 34-36.

Gospels, The Four.

LOWE, J. : Medical Missions. 1887. pp. 1-23, 147-164.

Medical Arm of the Missionary Service, The : 1898 p. 5.

Medical Missions at Home and Abroad: June, 1894, p. 133 ; Feb., 1896, p. 69.

Student Volunteer: Nov., 1897, p. 21.

WANLESS, W. J. : The Medical Mission. 1898. Chapters I. and II.

WILLIAMS, S. W. : The Middle Kingdom. 1895. Vol. I., p. 376 ; Vol. II., pp. 122, 123.

ADDITIONAL READINGS FOR CHAPTER II.

BALFOUR, EDW. : Cyclopedia of India. 1871-3. Article, Medicine.
BARNES, I. H. : Behind the Pardah. 1897. p. 178.
BRYSON, M. I. : John Kenneth Mackenzie (n. d.). pp. 287, 288.
CHRISTIE, DUGALD : Ten Years in Manchuria (n. d.). p. 85.
DENNIS, JAMES S. : Christian Missions and Social Progress. 1898.
Vol. I., pp. 102, 103, 110, 187-189, 192, 198, 207 210, 212.
Double Cross: May, 1896, p. 91.
DOWKONTT, GEO. D. : Murdered Millions. 1897 ed. pages 28-54.
LOWE, J. : Medical Missions. 1887. pp. 164-169.
Missionary Review of the World: Sept., 1895, pp. 679, 680, 688 ;
Sept., 1896, pp. 672-674 ; Feb , 1897, p. 159.
WANLESS, W. J. : The Medical Mission. 1898. Chapter III.
Women in Missions, p. 150.

ADDITIONAL READINGS FOR CHAPTER III.

British Medical Journal: Dec. 17, 1898, p. 1857.
BROWNING, ROBERT : Poem, The Strange Medical Experience of
Karshish.
BRYSON, M. I. : John Kenneth Mackenzie (n. d). p. 177.
Centenary Conference on Foreign Missions, London : 1888. Vol. I.,
p. 384.
DOWKONTT, GEO. D. : Murdered Millions. 1895. pp. 62-68, 74-86.
Encyclopedia of Missions : 1891. Vol. II., p. 52.
LOWE, J. : Medical Missions. 1887. pp. 171-174, 51-87 ; chapters
IV., V.
Medical Arm of the Missionary Service, The : 1898. pp. 35, 37-
40, 52.
Missionary Review of the World: Sept., 1895, p. 719.
PENNELL, T. L. : An Episode of the Afghan Medical Mission (n. d.).
pp. 1-12.
TRACY, C. C. : Talks on the Verandah. 1893. pp. 223, 224.
WANLESS, W. J. : The Medical Missions. 1898. Chapters IV.-VIII.
WANLESS, W. J. : Medical Missions, Facts and Testimonies.
WANLESS, W. J. : Medical Mission Work in India (n. d.).

ADDITIONAL READINGS FOR CHAPTER IV.

ACLAND, SIR HENRY : Medical Missions in relation to Oxford. 1898.
p. 27.
Centenary Conference on Foreign Missions, London, 1888. Vol. II.,
p. 110.
COLTMAN, R. : The Chinese. 1891. p. 175.
DENNIS, JAMES S. : Christian Missions and Social Progress. 1898.
Vol. I., pp. 120, 121, 125.
DOWKONTT, GEO. D. : Murdered Millions. 1895. pp. 86-88.
GRAVES, R. H. : Forty Years in China. 1895. pp. 237, 248.
LAURIE, T. : Missions and Science. 1885. pp. 125, 408, 411, 415.
LOWE, J. : Medical Missions. 1887. Chapter VII.
Medical Arm of the Missionary Service, The : 1898. pp. 52-54.
Woman in Missions, pp. 154, 156.

Bibliography

ADDITIONAL READINGS FOR CHAPTER V.

DOUGLAS. R. K. : Society in China. 1894. p. 152.
DENNIS, JAMES S. : Christian Missions and Social Progress. 1898.
Vol. I., pp. 120, 121.
FOSTER, A. : Christian Progress in China. 1889. p. 207.
Medical Arm of the Missionary Service, The : 1898. pp. 28, 29, 31.
Medical Missions at Home and Abroad : March, 1892, p. 86 ; June,
1894, p. 33.
Missionary Review of the World : Sept., 1895, p. 679.
Outlook : Sept., 1897, pp. 167-172.
THOBURN, J. M. : India and Malaysia. 1892. p. 384.
Women in Missions. pp. 160, 169.
WANLESS, W. J. : The Medical Mission. 1898. pp. 25-27.

ADDITIONAL READINGS FOR CHAPTER VI.

BEACH, H. P. : Dawn on the Hills of T'ang. 1898. pp. 117, 118.
Double Cross, The : May, 1896, p. 104 ; Sept., 1896, p. 187 ; July,
1898, p. 111 ; Sept., 1898, p. 145.
DOWKONTT, GEO. D. : Murdered Millions. 1895. pp. 12-19, 95, 96.
Isaiah, Chapter LXI.
LOWE, J. : Medical Missions. 1887. pp. 263-283.
Luke, Chapter XVI. 14-18.
Matthew, Chapter XXV. 31-46.
Medical Arm of the Missionary Service, The : 1898. pp. 12, 13.
Medical Missions at Home and Abroad : August, 1890, p. 164 ; Jan.,
1899, p. 235.
PHELPS, ELIZABETH STUART : The Story of Jesus Christ. 1898. pp.
135-160.
WANLESS, W. J. : The Medical Mission. 1898. Chapters X., XI.

www.ingramcontent.com/pod-product-compliance
Lightning Source LLC
Chambersburg PA
CBHW021828190326
41518CB00007B/786